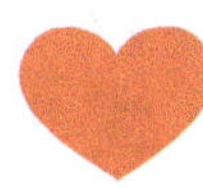

What people are saying about

NEVER EAT YOUR EMOTIONS AGAIN

Those of us who struggle with emotional eating know the journey to recovery is fraught with twists and turns, blind alleys, and harsh self-judgments. Marion's workbook series, *Never Eat Your Emotions Again,* provides readers with behavioral guidelines for success in that journey. She explores daily situations that can trigger the turn to food for comfort and exposes the mechanisms underneath. She offers readers means to achieve success in overcoming those pitfalls.

Marion's insider insights allow emotional eaters to feel understood and accepted, never judged. She creates strong connections with readers that allow them to re-establish contact with their own feelings and express what was numbed with food. This series is a needed complement to the growing literature on correct relationships to food.

Prof Oliver Morgan, Ph.D., LMFT, MAC

Author of Addiction, Attraction, Trauma, and Recovery
Clinical Fellow, AAMFT
Counseling & Human Services, University of Scranton

In *Never Eat Your Emotions Again,* Marion Holt illuminates the myriad factors that contribute to emotional eating and provides a road map to recovery. Emotional eating can have a negative effect on physical and mental health and often generates shame. This book provides an antidote to that shame by guiding the reader through an exploration of their emotional eating triggers and the process of developing effective strategies to mitigate and ultimately prevent it. As an obesity medicine specialist, I see how common emotional eating is and how it impacts the lives of those affected by it. *Never Eat Your Emotions Again* is a valuable resource for those who are ready to address their emotional eating and experience freedom and improved health.

Sandra Christensen, MSN, ARNP, FNP-BC, FOMA

Obesity Medicine Specialist, Obesity Medicine Association Board Trustee

Never Eat Your Emotions Again provides sound shadow work exercises to delve into the complexities of emotional overeating. Using her own personal stories and inner revelations, Marion Holt provides a safe space to explore the deepest recesses of our psyche without judgment or self-loathing.

Delving into the physical, mental, and relational manifestations of emotional eating exposes the layers of societal and/or familial conditioning we accept as our norm. This book provides the steps to reframe that narrative, freeing you to alter your mindset to challenge the "norm" and find peace with your true self.

Having the right mindset is the key to any success. Working with my own clients has taught me that without gaining and maintaining the successful mindset, it is far more difficult to achieve your goals. The techniques and exercises in this book provide guidance to obtaining that mindset. Working to change your relationship with food is a multitiered process that is well developed in this book.

Angela Atkins, INHC, CNT, CHt
Integrative Health & Nutrition Coach

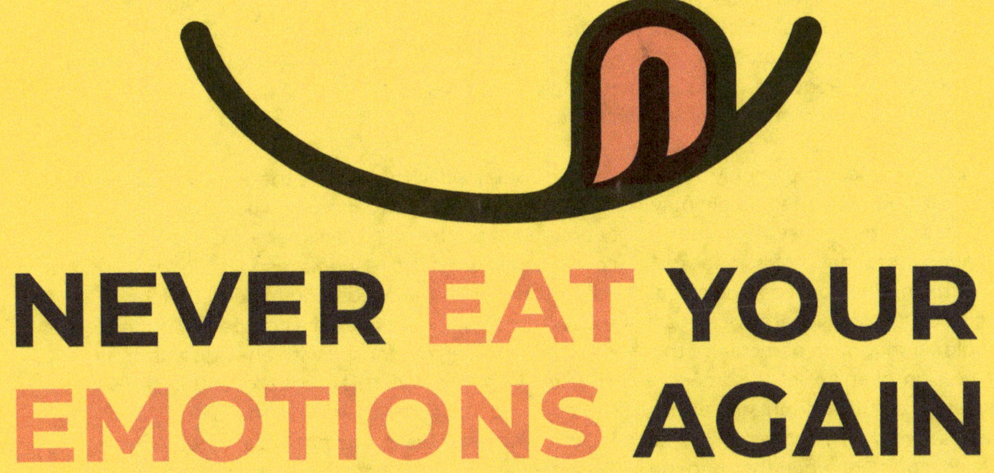

NEVER EAT YOUR EMOTIONS AGAIN

Breaking the Chain of Food Addiction

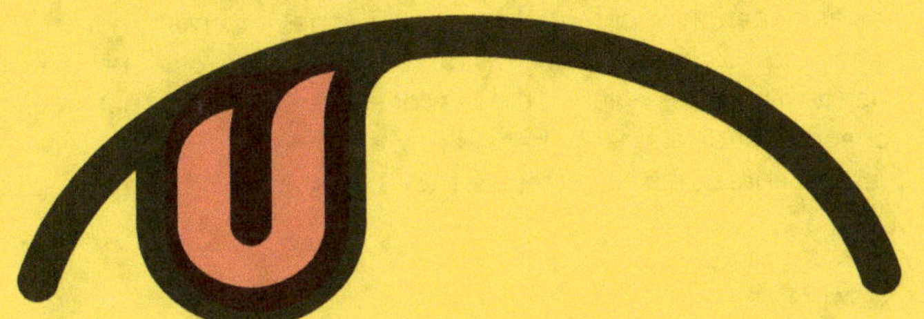

Marion Holt

NEVER EAT YOUR EMOTIONS AGAIN
Breaking the Chain of Food Addiction
© 2023 The Promise Within You, LLC

Disclaimer: For education only. The information contained in this book is the author's opinion. The strategies contained herein may not be suitable for every situation. This book is sold with the understanding that the author is not engaged in rendering medical, legal, psychological, nutritional, or other professional advice, counsel, or service. The reader is responsible for determining their own psychological, medical, and nutritional needs, and making their own decisions. If professional advice or assistance is required, the services of a competent professional should be sought. In particular, if the reader has ever been diagnosed with an eating disorder, depression, or an anxiety disorder, they agree to not go through this emotional eating recovery process without the input and approval of a psychiatrist, psychologist, or licensed dietitian. The reader also is responsible for their own and other eventual participants' safety, creating a safe environment when they engage in the activities proposed herein, ensuring that they, or anybody else, won't get hurt, and that there will be no material damage. If the reader cannot meet these requirements, they must not practice the activities proposed. The author shall not be liable for damages arising herefrom. The fact that an individual, organization, or website is referred to in this book as a citation or potential source of further information does not mean that the author endorses the information the individual, organization, or website may provide, or recommendations they/it may make. Further, the reader should be aware that websites listed in this book may have changed or disappeared between when this book was written and when it is read. If the reader does not agree with these terms, they are asked to not read the book.

ISBN (paperback): 979-8-9874188-0-2
ISBN (ebook): 979-8-9874188-1-9

Developmental Editing: Sandra Wendel; Copyediting: Candace Johnson
Proofreading: Michelle C. Booth
Cover Design and Interior Design: Anj Marie Riffel

Exercise in Step 3 inspired by *Presence* by Amy Cuddy, © 2014. Used with permission of Little, Brown Spark, an imprint of Hachette Book Group, Inc.

Published by The Promise Within You, LLC

Contact the author at: marion@nevereatyouremotionsagain.com

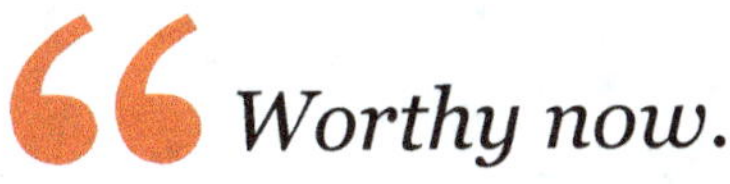 *Worthy now.*

Not if. Not when.

We are worthy of love and belonging now.

Right this minute.

As is."

— **Brené Brown**

CONTENTS

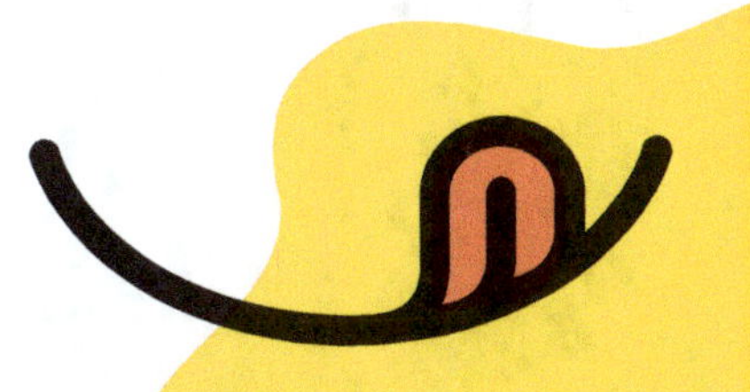

INTRODUCTION

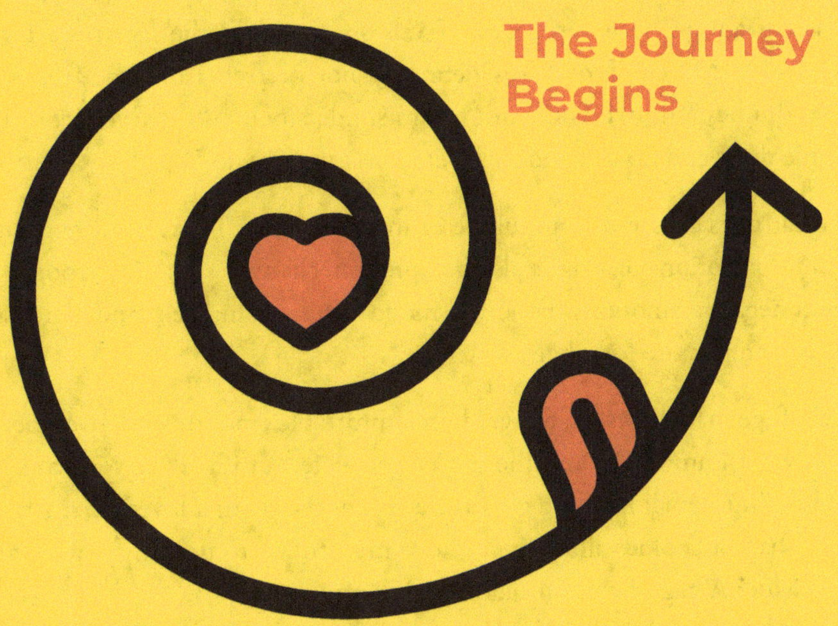

My Story

It is impossible for me to lose weight.

This is the story I used to tell myself. Afterall, why shouldn't I believe this? I had excellent reasons:

I have too much weight to lose.

My lifestyle is not compatible with a diet plan.

It simply never worked all the times that I have tried.

I know some have found a way, but there is no way for me.

My weight has always been a problem. I was six years old the first time I was placed on a diet. My childhood was definitely not perfect. Adulthood has not been either. But honestly, who does not feel misunderstood? Who never gets hurt? Many people don't end up affected by severe obesity. Why do I?

Emotional eating is a form of compulsive eating. I eat when I am not hungry, and I cannot stop. Emotional eating is also a coping mechanism. I eat in response to positive and negative emotions. Food is a mood regulator in itself, and I increase what I eat to compensate for what I feel.

Eating is a refuge that allows me to avoid uncomfortable emotions. My well-being depends on what I am eating and the size of my plate. A difficult day at work? A comfort-food dinner will help me get over it. A conflict with a loved one? An ice cream and a bag of cookies allow me to keep my cool. A restless night worrying about a life issue? A bag of chips usually soothes my anxiety.

Yes, I do gain weight because I eat too much and I don't move enough. Every expert I meet logically tells me that the solution is to eat less and move more. Duh. Wow! Like I never thought about it myself. The thing is: I can't. When cravings hit me, there is no way I can resist them, and no one provides me efficient guidance to solve that dilemma. I am alone with my pain—and with my shame.

I don't enjoy overeating. I don't like the way I feel when my cravings are finally satisfied and leave me alone, only to be replaced with guilt. I don't like being overweight. I tried many diet plans. Obeyed to the letter the advice of a dozen nutritionists. I left several sports coaches bald from pulling their hair out. I even went through bariatric surgery. I did lose some weight … for a while. And gained it all back, with some extra, just as quickly.

I learned several healthy ways of eating and safe ways to exercise. I know a ten-minute method to manage my anxiety. I am involved in several fun activities to keep from getting bored, and I own many weight loss meal plans. It is important, but it is not enough. These methods never worked for me.

To me, emotional eating feels like having a friend in my stomach. I start off with this friend, thinking they have my best interests in mind. They are going to help make my life better, and they are going to be there for me when other friends might not be. When in a really vulnerable position, I latch onto this friend. As I spend more time with them, I become bigger and bigger, and my life gets smaller and smaller. My friend gets meaner, and their demands get harder. Yet, I am trapped with them and feel as if I cannot survive without them. I can't let them go.

One day, I find myself basically as big as two people and living half a life, denying myself a lot of the experiences that would bring me happiness and joy. It's an awful way to live. It's a way so many of us live in silence, thinking maybe it is normal.

Today, I am not affected by obesity anymore.

I stopped treating food as the villain. I faced my issues for what they were and made the decisions I was scared to make. I am finally able to stick to a healthy lifestyle, not as a primary change but as a consequence of my emotional eating recovery. I face every new day without carrying the weight of years of untold pain buried under food. When something upsets me today, I just have to deal with today. There is nothing to silence anymore, nothing to hide, nothing to keep control of, no friend to appease. I am at peace. Inner peace makes it so much easier now to stay on track and keep making healthy choices.

What This Book Is and What It Is Not

Never Eat Your Emotions Again, **in three volumes, is not a diet book series.** Food is not the issue for us emotional eaters. Food is just the way we deal with our issues. It is what makes being alive bearable in spite of our issues. We won't discuss food, eating habits, or exercise here. At all.

🚫 **This is not a series about obesity.** Healthcare professionals talk about how obesity shortens life. They raise awareness about sugar and how it works like heroin in our brains. Most of the existing weight loss methods focus on the physical consequences of what makes us eat: our extra weight. We won't. We will focus on the primary issue that emotional eaters have to deal with, which is behavioral: why we eat when not hungry, and how to stop.

🚫 **This series is not a testimonial describing my weight loss journey nor the journal of my emotional eating recovery.** I do share elements of my own story when I believe it is useful to illustrate a specific point or to help you reflect on your own situation by analyzing mine. But this is not about me. It is about you.

🚫 **This series is not simply about intellectually understanding the mechanisms of emotional eating.** It is rooted in real life and is meant to help you bring some change in your everyday life. I will give you information, explanations, and technical knowledge about what is going on, from a behavioral point of view, when you eat your emotions. I will also ask you questions encouraging self-observation and propose activities to engage you.

🚫 **This series is not about finding better ways than eating to cope with our emotions.** We don't need to learn new ways to distract ourselves from what we feel. This series is about healing the pain we silence with food and adjusting our way of life so we don't need the comfort of food anymore.

🚫 **This series does not provide any generic truths or solutions that work for all of us. There will be no "3 easy steps" or "simple trick" to try.** I wish there was a universal answer to emotional eating, but we all use food as a coping mechanism for unique reasons and in very personal ways. This guide unfolds an introspective process and includes questions and training that are doors to discovering your own answers. Actual recovery will be your journey, but you don't have to make it alone. How you choose to answer these questions and go through these training exercises will bring lasting change to your life and transform your relationship with food.

Who Am I to Tell You What to Do?

As far as I can remember, I have always relied on food to be able to make it through the day without breaking down. I have always been overweight, and I was affected by severe obesity for much of my adult life. I reached out to everyone and tried everything I thought might help me, even the most exotic techniques. Unsuccessfully. I know exactly how it feels to be stuck there. I know life and its challenges as an overweight emotional eater because I was one most of my life.

I am a recovering emotional eater. I was stuck in my relationship with food. Then I changed. I have not studied emotional eating recovery in books. I did not follow some expert's directions. I wish I could have, but I didn't find any that were efficient for me. So I decided to stop relying on people who could not help me and to take back my own power. I learned by myself how emotional eating works and what I needed to do to get out. I experienced relapses and moments of despair. I made many mistakes and gained back all the weight I lost, then lost it again. I know the dead ends, I know the tricks our minds can play, and I know what works.

I was trained and certified as a professional behavior coach. I know how individuals get stuck in negative patterns, and I know how to get them out. I am used to understanding my clients' perspectives and bringing change into their lives. I have worked with emotional eaters, and I have witnessed some incredible transformations. I am able to connect my personal experience with emotional eating and my expertise in human behavior to build a recovery path.

The process I propose to you in this book is based on:

- my own experience of the challenges met as an emotional eater,
- my expertise as a professional behavior coach,
- my work with other emotional eaters, and
- my own emotional eating recovery.

When I Knew I Could Provide Efficient Help to Other Emotional Eaters

I was still affected by severe obesity when my first weight-loss coaching client chose me to work on their weight issues. I could not understand why they would want to work with me, as I had even more weight to lose than they did! They simply said, "I want to work with you precisely because you are overweight. I know you can understand me."

I indeed understood their point immediately. As I have since worked with many emotional eaters, it always strikes me how, even if our stories are different, our pain and how we deal with our wounds are the same.

In my own personal experience as an overweight person trying to lose weight and reaching out for professional help, I never felt understood. I went to doctors, nutritionists, dietitians, sports coaches, psychotherapists, and diet counselors. They were the experts, though it appeared none of them had weight issues. They did their best to help me, but their perception of what I was going through and what I needed to do to overcome my weight issues never matched my reality.

As I could never trust them to understand me, I never fully opened up either. I have discovered with my clients how simply being able to genuinely tell the truth about our situation makes a big difference. I will ask you to be real throughout this book because it is essential to a successful emotional eating recovery. I know how vulnerable it feels to open up totally and how difficult it can be, especially when we have not allowed ourselves to put our masks down for years, sometimes decades. I believe in leading by example, so I choose to open the way: I don't talk about my clients' experiences in this book; I talk about mine, as authentically as I can. Whenever you are unsure or uncomfortable, just follow my lead.

After my initial client lost over seventy pounds, I resolved to embark on my own weight loss journey. I applied to myself what I used during my work with clients— and more. I needed several years to process the emotional aspect of my weight issues and achieve a significant weight loss. During that time, I realized that many other people have issues losing weight because they also eat their emotions and don't know how to stop. Sometimes, they don't even know it's a thing and judge themselves badly for not being able to stick to a diet. So I decided to conceptualize an emotional eating recovery process and share it. This has now become the focus of my work.

Today, as I witness others facing the same issues as mine, I know laziness or lack of willpower are never at fault. When I see someone failing to lose weight or making unhealthy food choices, I wonder what situational factors are holding this person back. What needs are currently not being met? What are the pain and fear barriers to action that I cannot see? There are always barriers. Recognizing them and viewing those barriers as legitimate are often the first step in breaking "lazy" or "weak" behavior patterns on our path to recovery.

How to Read This Book

Like we would peel an onion, this guide in three volumes starts with the outer layers. Each chapter will take you closer to the heart of the matter. You can start reading here in book 1, step 1, and follow the path, digging a bit deeper at every step, until the last chapter of book 3. However, healing doesn't come in the same way for everybody. Some of us may be ready to face some emotional difficulties, while some may not be there yet but are able to face others. Some people may already have solved certain issues leading them to eat their emotions and already have adjusted some of their behaviors.

Recovering from emotional eating is a journey, and we all go through it in our own very personal way. This is why every chapter in all three volumes is independent of the next one, and you are free to enter the adventure by jumping directly to the chapters that appeal to you the most, whatever volume they are included in, navigating through every step at your pace and in the order that feels right to you. This series is for you and to help you.

Sometimes, though, our emotional resistance tricks us into believing that we are already through a specific matter or that this one issue simply doesn't apply to us. A part of you may subconsciously want to avoid digging too deeply into a topic and will decide it is pointless to explore in that direction because you secretly fear it might be hurtful. That's why I start every chapter with my personal experience. If my story finds any sort of echo in you, it might be worth digging into that chapter a bit further, even if you feel resistance—rather, *especially* if you feel resistance. There may be something important there for you to embrace so that you can heal or finish healing.

My real-life examples sometimes involve my parents. This does not mean that you have to systematically explore your relationship with your own parents or the people who raised you. It simply means that my own emotional eating is partially connected to my relationship with them.

What is important for you to consider is not the people involved in my stories or how old I was when some events occurred. Instead, please focus on the types of situations exposed and the emotions described. Determine if you have ever felt this way, too, or found yourself in a similar situation, regardless of who else was involved or your age when it happened.

This series maps a way out of emotional eating. It unfolds a recovery process and takes you through it. I don't know what you will discover during your journey. I don't have a universal solution that works for all of us. I will offer you guidance on how to approach every topic and to take every step of this journey; I will highlight possible blind spots in your thinking; and I will help you clarify some of your priorities, but I cannot point you to the *right* decision to make. The decision is yours.

In the same way, I don't know what your pace will be either. You may fly through some chapters in a couple of hours and need to spend weeks on others. That's okay. It's not a race. You've probably been stuck with emotional eating for quite some time, and if a few more weeks to process all that you have been going through are necessary, does it really matter? What is important is that you take the time you need to explore every aspect and heal.

This series is conceived as an alternative to counseling or therapy. Therefore, during the introspection proposed and because of the emotions associated with the deeper understanding you will gain about yourself, some elements of your past and the choices you made will sometimes feel like an emotional roller coaster. You will probably experience some low spots, followed by some exhilarating aha moments. Overall, this is not going to be an easy read, and it is important that you are prepared. You are about to unveil what you have been numbing and muting with food for a long time. And you would not have needed the help of food if it was easy to face. But I will be right there with you all the time.

In this book, you will see the highly effective techniques—role-playing, letter writing, visualizations, and powerful exercises—I use to take many of my clients from their painful relationship with food to the freeing realization that the pain and confusion they feel can be lifted. Some of our work in this book will be aimed at helping you accept some uncomfortable truths at the deepest levels of your being and fully acknowledging what has been going on in your life. Other parts of our work in this book will focus on how you can heal your head, your gut, and your heart—and make sound decisions about how to handle your relationship with food.

This work requires great courage and a willingness to enter parts of your inner world that, in some cases, hold lifelong pain, disappointments, fears, and anger. I will ask you some questions that you may find confronting. I will also point out some truths that may feel uncomfortable. Please remember: every tough question I ask you, I asked myself first. Every uncomfortable truth, I had to embrace too. Every proposed activity, I went through it also. I absolutely know how it feels. I know it can be difficult sometimes. I also know it is necessary, and it is all worth it. Bravely acknowledging this material and bringing it to the bright light of consciousness will drain its power over you, and the liberation that results can be life-changing. Once you have the courage to accept the truth, you can free yourself from the wounds that have made you turn to food.

When and if some aspects or questions get too triggering for you, it is okay to put the book down for a little while and take a breather. Go at your own pace. Read a little of this book, then take the time to let what you have read sink in before going on. Don't try to stuff your feelings. You will probably cry a lot—and that's fine. Grief and anger are a natural, necessary part of this process. What is important is to keep moving forward—do not quit. Take a break if and when necessary, then come back.

Please, keep in mind that all your emotions are always welcome at every step of this journey.

✓   **It is okay to be sad.**

✓   **It is okay to be angry.**

✓   **And it is okay to be scared.**

Please keep in mind that the exercises in this book are not intended to replace in-person work with therapists, support groups, or twelve-step programs. I encourage you to reach out to a professional and get support if you feel overwhelmed. It is important that you have someone to turn to as you embark on this journey. If a severe trauma has influenced your relationship with food, it is *imperative* that you get professional help. Seeking help is a sign of strength, not weakness.

Some Guidelines for Choosing a Good Therapist

If you decide you'd like the help of a therapist, be sure the person you are going to work with is comfortable and experienced in dealing with unhealthy relationships with food and the emotional damages that lead to it.

Please don't stay with a therapist who hears your history and says things like

- That's all in the past—you need to move on.
- Let's just deal with the here and now.
- You don't want to spend your life feeling sorry for yourself.
- What (this person) told you/did to you many years ago does not impact what you put in your mouth today.

All these comments are dismissive, and they discount your feelings and experience. Working with a person who approaches your situation that way will only confuse and frustrate you, further reinforcing the self-blame you may already feel. ("Why am I being so weak-willed/lazy around food?" "Why can't I just stick to a diet like anybody else?")

Look for a therapist who works actively with you instead of just sitting back and saying, "Uh-huh" or "How do you feel about that?" You want a person who gives you feedback and actively engages with you. Trust your instincts. If you don't feel comfortable, safe, or truly heard when you are with your therapist, he or she is not the person for you.

From my own experience and those of the many others I've helped, I can tell you it is possible to change the belief that you cannot lose weight, and achieve a significant, long-lasting weight loss. I promise you that as we work together in this book, you will gain a wonderful sense of wholeness. In yourself and the world around you, you will find paths to the self-love, self-respect, hope, empowerment, and caring that you've craved for so long. There is an end to silence, there is an end to loneliness, and there is an end to pain. Let's break the chains and get your freedom back, together.

This book is intended to be your companion through your recovery journey. You can return to its content again and again for guidance, validation, and support. You are not alone in this. Ask for help anytime. The emotional path I am taking you on is difficult, and I am aware of that. You might also find some insight and additional emotional support from others who truly understand your journey on my free Facebook Support Group.

< You can join here

Never Eat Your Emotions Again Network

www.facebook.com/groups/nevereatyouremotionsagain

Whether you're just starting out on your journey and need some advice, or you've been at this a while and are stuck, email or message me. Make sure to sign up for my free email newsletter that gives monthly tips to help you be successful during your journey. Think of me as your weight loss buddy. We are partners, and we are facing this together. I am with you, and I am going to stick with you. Even if you cannot see it right now, there is a way out. I have made it to the other side, and you will too.

Let the journey begin!

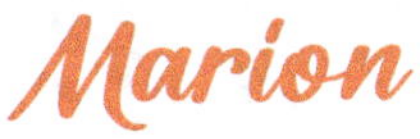

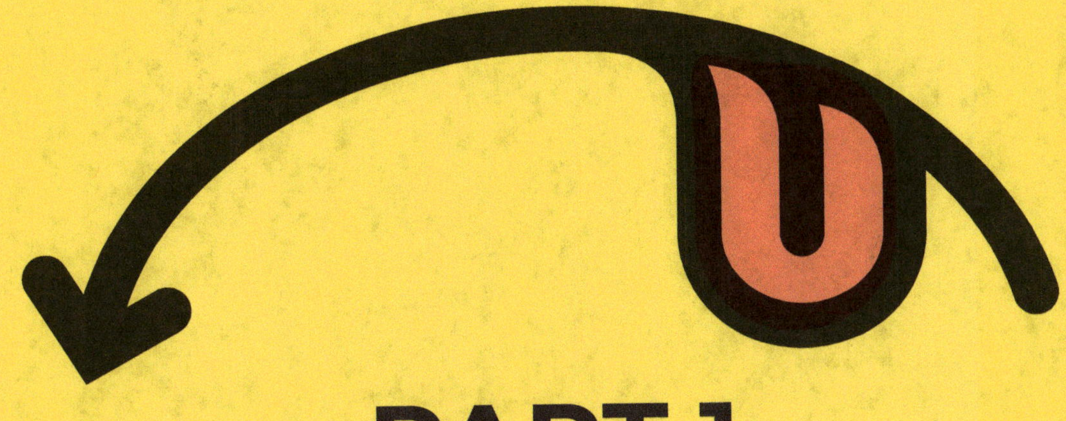

PART 1

From a Negative to a Positive Perception of Yourself

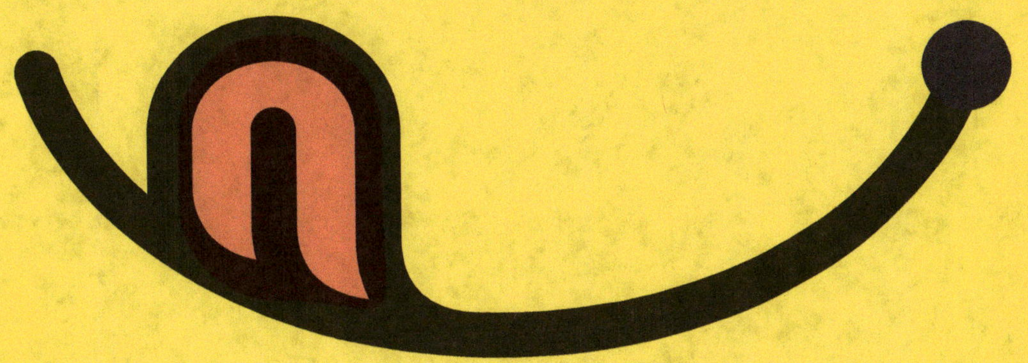

Change Your Mind

You Can Lose Weight

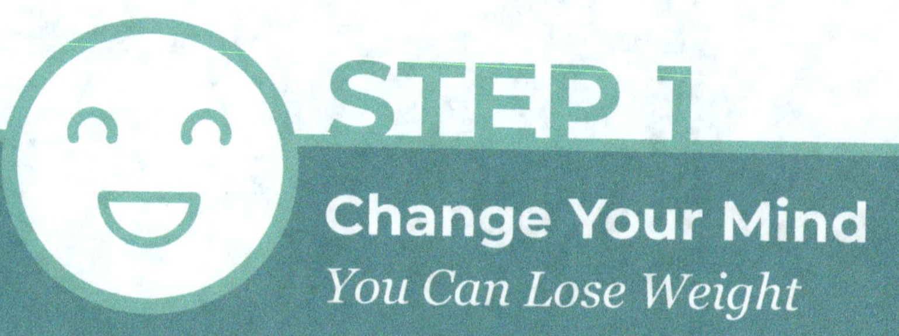

STEP 1

Change Your Mind
You Can Lose Weight

When I start watching my diet, I have a positive attitude.
I feel motivated, and I believe I can be successful. Over time, it gets harder to resist my urge to eat. When something difficult occurs in my life, I *need* to eat in order to calm down, and I come to the realization that I simply cannot do this: I am unable to change.

I am unhappy. I am overweight, and it prevents me from enjoying myself and being who I want to be. My extra weight is the one thing that continues to mess up my entire life. I would give anything to be "normal." People tell me I don't really want to lose weight. They say I find excuses not to lose weight.

Truth is: I want to, but I don't believe I can. And the best proof lies in how often I tried. I have tried so many times and failed every time. It's a losing battle. I have lost hope. I cannot lose weight. I don't see anything or anyone who can really help me. I cannot think of anything that can keep me motivated to keep up with my diet when it gets really tough. I am simply not strong enough.

There are a thousand good reasons that make it difficult for me to lose weight, yet I fail to find a single one that truly encourages me to push through. I focus on why I gained weight in the past and why I cannot lose weight today. As I don't truly believe I have the ability to lose weight, I am bitter, and I complain. I focus on what went wrong in my life and the guilty people, past events, toxic relationships, judgmental professionals, impossible social standards, and the food advertisers who trick me into buying products loaded with hidden sugar and carbohydrates. Why would I totally commit and do everything I can to lose weight when I don't really believe that I can?

As I don't believe that I can lose weight, my life feels more enjoyable with comfort food that tastes good than without. I believe that comfort food makes my life more fulfilled than healthy food. I believe if I switch to healthy food, I will be sadder, my life will end up less appealing, and I will not lose weight anyway.

I constantly postpone the decision to try to lose weight for fear of not being able to live a fulfilled life. I risk dying early for the illusion of living a rewarded life. But I do not live a fulfilled life when I spend my weekends as a couch potato, alone, eating junk food, and binge-watching television shows. Wow. This sure is not the life I dreamed about. My current situation simply does not allow me more. I am well on my way to dying young and unhappy because I believe that I cannot lose weight and that a weekend alone on the couch is fulfilling. I don't live; I just kill time the best I can because I believe I cannot expect anything more from my life.

As long as I don't address my beliefs, I don't try to change. I simply trick myself into believing that I am trying every time I go on a new diet. I prepare the ground for my own failure, and I reinforce the belief that I cannot lose weight, building the wall of truth every time. Until I don't even try anymore. When I constantly focus on the logical, pragmatic, irrefutable reasons why it is impossible for me to lose weight, why would I even try to put effort into an impossible change?

If I cannot lose weight today, it is because *today*, I absolutely don't believe I can.

But what if I decide that I can? What if I believe that it is worth trying, for real this time? How do I evolve from focusing on negative justifications to positive, supportive, and helpful thoughts? How do I transform my relationship with food and with my body? How do I let go of my negative beliefs and start looking for what I truly need?

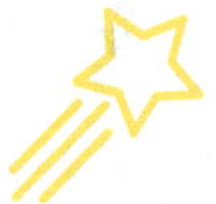# The Challenge: Limiting Beliefs

We all have beliefs grounded in fact and beliefs rooted in emotion and life experience. These belief systems shape how we view the world and ourselves. Louise Hay says, "We learn our belief systems as very little children, and then we move through life creating experiences to match our beliefs. Look back in your own life and notice how often you have gone through the same experience."

Beliefs are essentially assumptions we make about ourselves, about others, and about how we expect things to be in our world. We have theories, ideas, and explanations about how things are and how they ought to be. We draw conclusions about life, ourselves, and other people, all of which help us make better sense of the world. Beliefs form the foundation of our expectations. These expectations help us better understand ourselves and others and the world around us. They help us feel more certain about the future, which makes us feel safe and secure.

Beliefs certainly are not facts, even if they can sometimes be mistaken for facts. They simply are conclusions we have drawn. Many of our beliefs were ingrained in our brains as children, and they often came from our parents and other influential adults. In most cases, these beliefs serve us well up to a certain point. But after that point, some beliefs become limiting and sometimes even damaging.

Limiting beliefs constrain us in some way. Just by believing them, we do not think, do, or say the things they inhibit.

Statements of Limiting Beliefs

I do/I don't. We often judge ourselves in negative ways. Some of us may define ourselves by what we deserve or do not deserve. When we think, "I don't deserve" to be slimmer, happy, or loved, then we do not expect or seek happiness, love, or ways to become healthier.

I can/I can't. We often have limited self-images of what we can and cannot do. Some of us may believe that our abilities are fixed and that we cannot learn. If we think, "I cannot lose weight," then we will stop trying.

I must/I mustn't. We are bound by values, norms, laws, and other rules that constrain what we must and must not do. However, not all of these are mandatory, and some are distinctly limiting. If we think, "I must hide my feelings," this takes away the chance to express them and contributes to creating our need to eat them.

I am/I am not. The use of the verb *to be* can be harmful, because as we think, "I am," we also think, "I am not" or "I cannot." When we think, "I am fat," it may mean that fat is a part of what we are, so we conclude that we can never get fit or slim or be able to exercise. "I am" thinking assumes we cannot change.

Others are/Others will. Just as we have limiting beliefs about ourselves, we also have beliefs about other people, which can limit us in many ways. If we think others are more capable and superior to us, then we will not be able to have balanced relationships with them. We guess what others are thinking based on our beliefs about them. We may believe they do not like us when they actually have no particular opinion, or even think we are rather nice. We then deduce their likely actions, which can be completely wrong.

Why We Limit Our Beliefs

We create limitations in our beliefs in a variety of ways.

Experience. A key way by which we all form our beliefs is through our direct experiences. We act, something happens, and we draw conclusions. Such beliefs are often helpful, but they can also be limiting. We learn and build beliefs faster from harmful experiences. For example, sticking a finger on a hot stove hurts a lot, so we believe all stoves are dangerous and never touch a stove again. This is a helpful belief. But when we go on a diet, fail to lose weight, and draw the conclusion that we are not able to lose weight, we create a harmful belief.

Education. When forming our perceptions of the world, we cannot depend on experience for everything. Hence, we read and listen to our parents, authority figures, and teachers about how the world works and how to conduct ourselves. But our teachers are not always well informed. We also learn from what peers tell us, but they are limited by their own beliefs, which they transmit to us.

Education is a double-edged sword. It tells us what is right and wrong, good and bad. It helps us survive and grow, but just because we were told something, we may never try things and so miss pleasant, useful experiences and knowledge. For example, I might want to become a flight attendant but have the perception I need to be fit in order to be hired for that type of position. As I am overweight, I do not even send my application and get a ground job instead. In spite of what I was told, I see many plump flight attendants on planes when I travel, and I could have been hired.

Excuse. Sometimes, we form limiting beliefs to excuse ourselves from what we perceive to be our failures. When we do something that does not work, we may explain away our failure by forming and using beliefs that justify our actions and leave us blameless. In doing so, we do not learn from our failures, and we cannot grow. We avoid taking responsibility for our failed attempts. But if it is "not my fault," there is nothing we can do to avoid failing the next time we try. Success or failure does not depend on what we do or stop doing. This mindset may lead us to increasingly paint ourselves into a corner, limiting what we will think and do in the future. For example, "I cannot stop eating at 6:00 p.m. because I am unable to sleep when I go to bed hungry." Or, "I have no sense of discipline, and I am unable to stop eating after just one cookie or one bag of cookies."

Fear. Limiting beliefs can also be fear-driven. We may think if we go against some of our beliefs, some of our needs will be harmed. There is often a social component to our decisions, and the thought of criticism, ridicule, or rejection by others is enough to powerfully inhibit us. We also fear that we may be harmed in some way by others, so we avoid them or seek to appease them.

For example, "If I lose weight and become attractive, my friends may see me as competition and reject me." What really hides behind our fear of becoming more attractive? Is it the possibility that someone will have a desire for us and all the associated emotions that go along with that? Is it the fear of being vulnerable? The fear of a possible rejection? Something else?

How to Get Rid of Your Limiting Beliefs

There is predictive power in what we believe: what we believe in usually ends up happening. Some call this a *self-fulfilling prophecy.* For example, if I believe that I will never fit into a size ten, I can be sure that, indeed, I never will. A belief is what we think is right, whether we are aware we believe so or not. The power of our beliefs has influenced our personality and our behaviors and has shaped our reality. Beliefs shape our future and our personal story. Some are positive and feed our sense of personal efficacy. Some are negative and drain our energy, making it impossible to even start moving toward weight loss.

When it comes to our ability to lose weight, our negative beliefs are usually constructed on our past failures; because we failed to consistently lose weight before, we believe we cannot succeed today. But your future is not defined by your past. Today, you can choose to believe you can lose weight.

 *Identify Your Limiting Beliefs*

If your goal is to change something, the first step is to identify what you are dealing with. Let's start with acknowledging how challenged you may feel with your current life and your current relationship with food. Please consider your health and your relationships and how much you enjoy life, and evaluate how you are doing in these areas.

Health. On a sliding scale from 1 to 10, 1 for not at all and 10 for extremely, how much do you take care of your health? *(Do you go to the doctor when you are sick? Do you pay attention and treat physical discomforts like skin rash, toothaches, back issues, joint issues, or small wounds? Do you have a physical examination every year? Do you wear comfortable clothes/underwear? Do you wear comfortable and adapted shoes and buy a new pair when they do not provide good support anymore?)*

1   2   3   4   5   6   7   8   9   10

Relationships. On a sliding scale from 1 to 10, 1 for not at all and 10 for extremely, how satisfying are your relationships? *(Please consider your intimate relationship as well as your relationships with your family, friends, and coworkers.)*

1   2   3   4   5   6   7   8   9   10

Fun and Adventure. On a sliding scale from 1 to 10, 1 for almost never and 10 for very often, how often are you doing the activities you really want to do? *(Hobbies, vacations, outdoor activities, reunions, and the like)*

1   2   3   4   5   6   7   8   9   10

Food. On a sliding scale from 1 to 10, 1 for not at all and 10 for extremely, how much is your relationship with food a factor of well-being or unease in these three areas? *(health, relationships, and fun)*

1 2 3 4 5 6 7 8 9 10

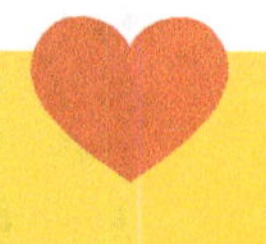

If you are not happy with your life in general or specifically your weight and way of eating, and you are not actively doing something to change, then you probably have one or several limiting beliefs.

➜ **What negative statements do you make about yourself?**

____

____

➜ **What negative statements do you make to yourself about your ability to lose weight?**

____

____

➜ **What negative statements do you make to yourself about your lovability?**

____

____

➜ **Where have you heard those statements before? Whose voice is this?** *(Is this the voice of a parent, relative, sibling, friend, teacher, minister, priest, or coach? Are these statements you have heard from society? Is the voice imagined or real?)*

____

____

Our internal world is where beliefs are created. Here are a few of my own negative beliefs about myself, my life in general, and my relationship with food. Please check the ones that you share with me, and add the beliefs that impact you and are not listed. You may have limiting beliefs about your rights, your duties, your abilities, or your permissions. Please write down everything that comes to mind.

- ☐ It is impossible for me to lose weight.
- ☐ One cannot have it all in life.
- ☐ Losing weight is extremely difficult for anybody.
- ☐ I am too old to lose weight. It's too late.
- ☐ To be loved by other people, I must please them.
  To be loved, I must earn it.
- ☐ I do not deserve to be happy.
- ☐ Getting out of obesity is just a dream; it's too good to be true.
- ☐ I cannot afford to make a mistake.
- ☐ Being imperfect is a failure.
- ☐ Happiness is not at hand.
- ☐ I will never make it.
- ☐ If I am fit, I will become pretentious and shallow.
- ☐ If I am attractive, abusers will prey on me.
- ☐ I must reach that precise weight at that precise time.
- ☐ I am affected by obesity because I had a difficult childhood.
- ☐ I am affected by obesity because a few years ago, a bad injury/a pregnancy/a medical condition kept me inactive for a while, and I put on a lot of weight at that time.
- ☐ Constantly watching what I eat is not compatible with my lifestyle.
- ☐ The food I am given doesn't allow me to lose weight.
- ☐ I do not belong in a gym.
- ☐ I do not have time to cook.
- ☐ I am not able to watch what I eat for months (or years).
- ☐ I have a slow metabolism.
- ☐ I must be fit to live a happy life.

☐ I need an accountability buddy in my weight loss process.

☐ If I lose weight, I will end up with loose skin and stretch marks, and it is going to be just as bad as being fat, maybe worse.

☐ Losing weight is only a matter of willpower. As I stay fat, I have no willpower.

☐ I will get on a diet when I get better, happier, or when I find a boyfriend who loves me.

☐ Everything is in my head. My extra pounds will disappear by themselves as soon as I am more fulfilled.

☐ It's not my fault. When life gets easier, I will naturally eat less.

☐ Eating healthy food is more expensive than eating junk food. I cannot afford to eat healthy food.

☐ I can do this on my own, without telling anybody.

☐ I am affected by obesity, but all is good.

☐ I am affected by obesity, but I am in good health.

☐ I am fat, but I love my body just the way it is.

☐ I gained weight after some traumatic events, and now I am stuck in this body.

☐ I do not like vegetables. They do not taste good.

☐ I do not like the taste of plain water.

☐ I do not want to give up food; it is my only source of enjoyment in life.

☐ My environment sabotages all my efforts.

☐ My knee/hip/back hurts, and I cannot exercise.

☐ I work night shifts; I cannot be on a diet.

☐ I have no self-control.

☐ I need motivation before I am able to get on a diet.

☐ Fit people do not need to watch what they eat to stay fit. It is just my bad luck.

☐ If I cut my food intake, I will switch to starvation mode, and I will end up gaining weight.

☐ Nothing I do works.

☐ I am lazy, and I like being a couch potato.

☐ I don't have the equipment I need to exercise correctly.

☐   I am just too busy. I don't have the time.

☐   My weight is my protection.

☐   My weight is a part of my identity.

☐   I am going through menopause; it is too late to lose weight.

____

____

____

____

____

____

____

→ On a sliding scale from 1 to 10, 1 for not significant at all and 10 for extremely, how significant is the impact of these beliefs on your emotional eating?

1   2   3   4   5   6   7   8   9   10

→ How does believing these affirmations contribute to your emotional eating?

____

____

You are doing great! Limiting beliefs can be especially difficult to spot because they sneak into our thoughts without us being aware of them. Before we know it, they have become "the truth" in our mind. But don't believe everything you think. Just because you thought it doesn't make it legitimate.

 ## *Eliminate Your Limiting Beliefs*

→ **What do you think about your emotional eating and your current situation?**
(relationship with food, body shape, body image)

____

____

____

→ **How do you label yourself when it comes to emotional eating and your ability to overcome it?**

____

____

____

→ **What specifically gets in your way when you try to stop eating your emotions?**

____

____

____

→ **What makes you think this obstacle is too difficult to overcome?**

____

____

____

→ **What specific beliefs are holding you back right now?**

These are all wrong. They hurt you, and they limit you. It is time to stop carrying them.

Please take a piece of paper and write down these limiting beliefs. When you are done, destroy that piece of paper in the way that you decide is the most appropriate: You can go for a walk and bury it in the ground. You can burn it, flush it down the toilet, cut it into pieces, tear it up. The most important thing is that the method you choose feels right to you. When you are done, simply state, "You are not true. I choose not to believe you anymore."

→ **Consider how your behavior can change now that you have eliminated these beliefs from your life. What can you do differently? How do these changes impact your emotional eating?**

Please, be kind with yourself. You have dealt with these negative beliefs for a long time, and erasing them will not happen overnight. When you get caught up in one, it does not mean you are failing; it simply means it is not easy to let it go. Just acknowledge the belief, and as you become more and more aware of it, it will be easier to fight its influence until it disappears.

 ## *Create New Beliefs That Serve You*

Once we take power away from our negative beliefs, we regain the ability to change and transform our limiting beliefs into positive ones.

Please write down the limiting beliefs that hold you back the most and have the greatest negative impact on your emotional eating. Next to each negative statement, write an opposite, positive affirmation.

NEGATIVE STATEMENT	POSITIVE AFFIRMATION
I am so terrible; I do not deserve to be loved by anyone.	*I am lovable just the way I am and deserve all the love in the world.*
✖	✓
✖	✓
✖	✓
✖	✓
✖	✓
✖	✓

Stating positive affirmations is one thing; believing in them is another. To turn these positive affirmations into your new beliefs, please imagine you want to explain the accuracy of these new beliefs to your best friend. What would you say? What point would you make to convince them that your new beliefs are true?

NEW BELIEF	WHY IT IS ACCURATE
I am lovable just the way I am, and I deserve all the love in the world.	*I deserve love because we all do. I am entitled to be loved as much as anyone else. I am generous and kind, and I always try to help others.*
✓	✓
✓	✓
✓	✓
✓	✓
✓	✓
✓	✓

We all carry numerous limiting beliefs. They come from a variety of sources as well as from our own interpretation of the world around us. Sometimes life teaches us things that are inaccurate. When we become aware of them, we have a choice; we can believe them or disregard them. Disregarding our beliefs takes awareness. We often do not realize every thought that pops into our minds is not true.

In the coming days, please try to raise your awareness about your thoughts. Every time you catch a negative belief popping into your mind, take control and choose to push it away. Tell yourself this is not the truth, and replace it with a positive belief. Use these new positive affirmations whenever the old limiting beliefs appear in your thoughts. The more you practice, the less often the limiting beliefs will show up until they simply cease to exist.

Jump-Start

→ How does your relationship with food influence your health?

____

____

____

→ How does your relationship with food influence your relationships with others?

____

____

____

→ How does your relationship with food influence the fun and adventure you have in life?

____

____

____

→ On a sliding scale from 1 to 10, 1 for not at all and 10 for very much, how much do you want to change your relationship with food today?

1   2   3   4   5   6   7   8   9   10

→ On a sliding scale from 1 to 10, 1 for not at all and 10 for very much, how much do you believe you can stop eating your emotions today?

1   2   3   4   5   6   7   8   9   10

Thinking Outside the Box

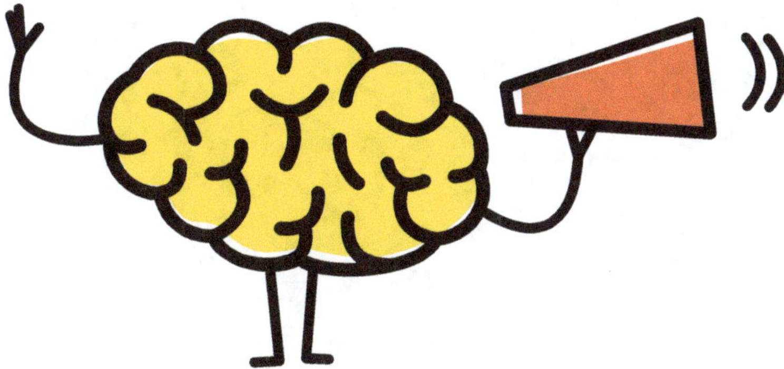

Most of us are familiar with this inner voice that tells us we are not good enough and undermines our accomplishments: "You're so unattractive. You're fat. What a slob. Just look at your hair, hips, waistline, beer belly." Our critical inner voice is formed from painful, early life experiences that we witnessed or came up against, or from hurtful attitudes toward us or those close to us. As we grow up, we unconsciously adopt and integrate this pattern of destructive thoughts toward ourselves.

When we fail to identify and separate ourselves from this inner critic, we allow it to impact our behavior and shape the direction of our lives. It may sabotage our successes or our relationships, preventing us from living the lives we want to lead and becoming the people we seek to be.

This is a coaching exercise meant to help you identify and overcome your critical inner voice. This voice builds your internalized dialogue, fosters self-criticism, and affects your self-esteem and inner confidence.

Please make sure you can have some quiet and alone time, in a safe environment, for the next twenty to thirty minutes. Get a pen or a few pencils. You can use the space available below or get a separate sheet of paper.

Draw a picture of the critical voice in your mind. It does not have to be artwork, and it does not need to be figurative. It can be an abstract drawing. There is no right or wrong. Just express how this critical voice feels to you without using words. Know this picture represents fears and judgments given to you but which do not belong to you.

→ As you are drawing, what thoughts are going through you? How are you feeling? What sensations are you experiencing?

Please take the time to look at your drawing for a while. You may want to change your perspective, turn it upside down, come closer to it or walk farther away, or adjust the intensity of light in the room.

➜ **What do you see?**

____

____

____

____

➜ **Where does this voice come from? What is the source of the voice attacks?**
(Do you recognize the content and tone of the voice attacks? Do they sound familiar? Does the voice say something someone around you used to tell you? Do the attacks give you the same feelings you got from someone else in the past? Do they remind you about something you experienced?)

____

____

____

____

➜ **Can you give the voice a name? What would it be?**

____

____

____

____

Please imagine speaking to your inner critical voice, the one that tells you all these negative beliefs and that makes all these negative statements about you. Ask it what it wants.

➔ **What is its intention?** *(Example: is this inner voice trying to protect or harm you?)*

➔ **What answer can you give to the voice? How do you shut it up?**

➔ **What positive statement(s) can you make about yourself in response to the voice attacks?**

The more we challenge our critical inner voice, the more we can recognize its limiting statements and where those statement come from, and then we can adjust them to serve us rather than hurt us.

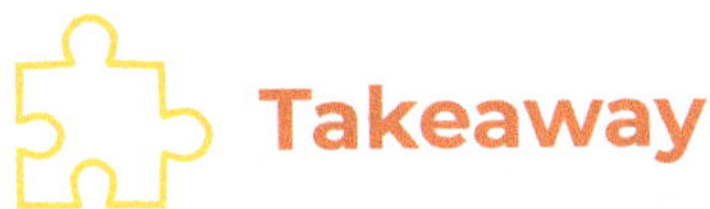

Takeaway

> *Man often becomes what he believes himself to be. If I keep on saying to myself that I cannot do a certain thing, it is possible that I may end by really becoming incapable of doing it. On the contrary, if I have the belief that I can do it, I shall surely acquire the capacity to do it even if I may not have it at the beginning."*
>
> —*Mahatma Gandhi*

You are already successful!

Congratulations! You made it through this important step. It was tough, but you pushed through it. Every time you engage in negative self-talk, please remember you've come this far, and there is no way you could have done this without willpower or a strong desire to bring positive and long-lasting change to your life.

In addition, you are probably not a total stranger to what we discussed in this chapter. That means you have been on your way to recovery for some time. Let's capitalize on your existing achievements and experience.

→ **What have you already tried/started/accomplished in the area discussed in this chapter that previously worked/was a success/was promising?**

____

____

____

→ **What happened to get you started?**

____

____

____

➜ **What was your recipe for success?**

➜ **How can you use this proven successful recipe today?**

Along the Path

➜ **What have you been through while reading this chapter?** *(What happened, how did you feel, what were your reactions, what important conversation did you have, did you have unusual dreams or body reactions/sensations?)*

➜ **What new perspective did you grasp in your relationship with food and with yourself or others or both?**

→ **What new concept did you discover?**

→ **What did you learn?**

→ **What realization did you come to?**

→ **What do you want to remember?**

Moving Forward

WHAT WILL YOU DO LESS?

✗

✗

✗

WHAT WILL YOU STOP DOING?

✗

✗

✗

WHAT WILL YOU START DOING?

✓

✓

✓

WHAT WILL YOU DO MORE OF?

✓

✓

✓

→ **Which one of these decisions will be the easiest for you to apply right now?**

You may feel what you have discovered or processed in this chapter is enough for you to successfully impact your relationship with food. If so, this is great, and you are ready to jump into the next change. You may also feel that it would be useful for you to dig deeper and explore these topics or some related areas a bit more. If you want to take your reflection process and experimentation one step further, do this exercise.

WHAT ASPECTS DO YOU WANT TO EXPLORE MORE?

HOW WILL YOU MAKE THIS EXPLORATION POSSIBLE?

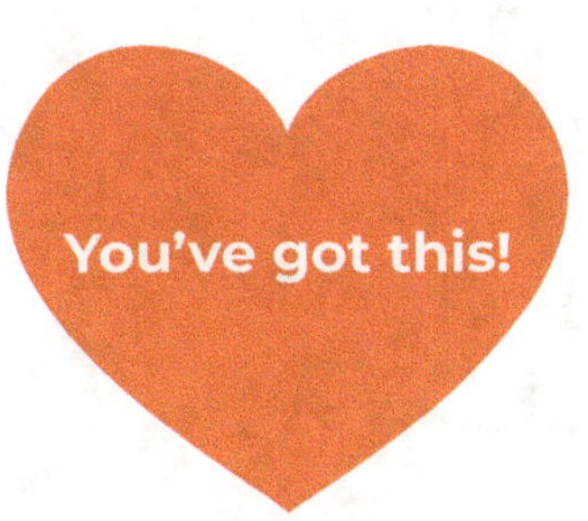

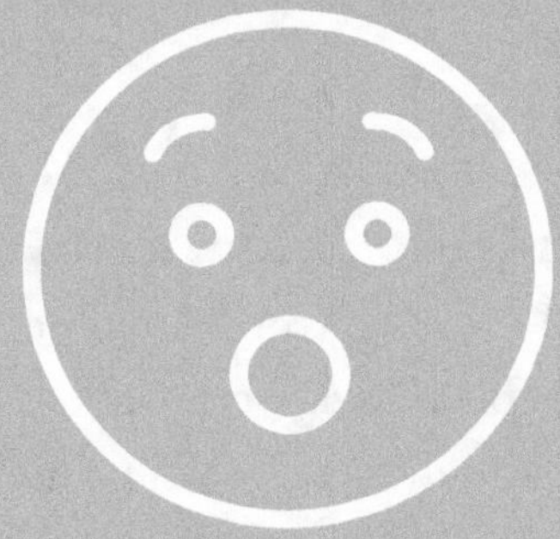

Cast Your Fears Away

You Can Change Even if Change Scares You

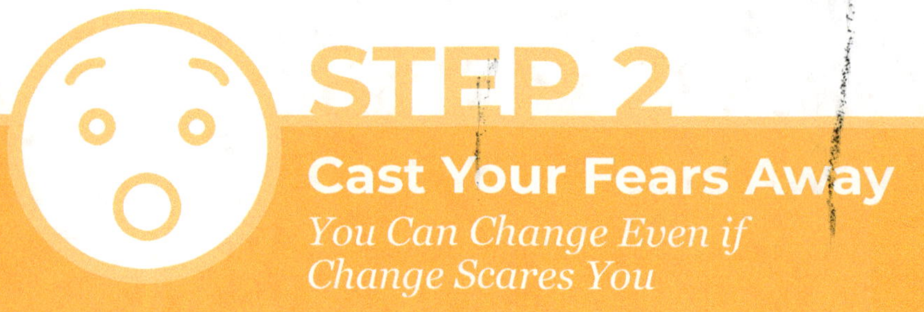

STEP 2

Cast Your Fears Away

You Can Change Even if Change Scares You

I have wanted to lose weight so badly for so long, and I've tried so hard, but time and again, I end up failing miserably. I set goals and objectives I just don't or cannot reach. I wonder why I keep repeating the same patterns of behavior over and over again and keep getting precisely the same frustrating results. I regret some things I did and some I did not do. Sometimes, I feel like I am my own worst enemy. I feel as if I have two minds: one that wants to lose weight and one that won't let me do it. There is always somebody (myself or others) standing in my way, and I can't resist them.

When I decide to lose weight, I usually start well.

My weight goes down at a satisfying pace. I am motivated enough to exercise several times a week and to stay on track. I can contemplate my weight goal, and I can start thinking it actually is attainable. Then something happens, and I revert to my old eating habits. Sometimes I am good during the day, but at night I start grazing and picking. I promise myself I will start watching my food intakes again the next morning, but I don't. Other times, I have a bad eating day. I instantly lose all motivation, then think I might as well quit, so I do. Sometimes I get back to my old patterns quickly, and sometimes they sneak up on me. But I am disappointed in myself every time, and that makes my next attempt to straighten out my relationship with food harder to get started. Until the day I simply give up completely.

A part of me doesn't want to lose weight and needs me to keep eating. This side of me believes I need to be strong, to be physically impressive and able to defend myself should I ever be threatened or attacked. This side of me believes being heavy means being strong. As a child, I had to accept many hurtful situations imposed by adults. I was not strong enough to oppose. When I tried to avoid doing what they wanted me to do, I was threatened and physically forced to do it anyway. As I was just a child, there was no way I could defend myself.

Being heavy today means I am physically strong. When I slap, I will hurt more than the slap I got. Being heavy today also means that anybody who bumps into me or shakes me up will be the one dealing with the kinetic energy released. I will not move, and they will receive the impact of the resistance. Today, I cannot be forcibly compelled to do something by anyone, and that makes me feel safe. If I lose my extra weight, I also lose this advantage, and I am terrified to be back in my powerless state where I just have to endure what stronger people do to me.

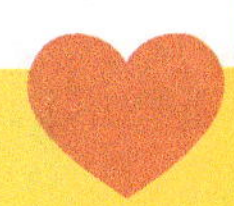

While one side of me tries to stop eating when not hungry, the other side fights to keep me heavy.

Sometimes, I also feel like others try to sabotage my efforts. Some people in my life try to belittle or undermine my weight loss efforts. My friends, coworkers, or family members tempt me with foods they know I am avoiding, while saying things like, "Just one bite won't hurt you," "You have come so far, you deserve to have just one little treat!" "I made this dish, you have to try it," or "It is my birthday, you have to have cake!"

People around me don't like that I suddenly turn from eating anything at any time to becoming picky and reading every food label. They cook and eat tempting food around me at every meal and offer me a box of my favorite chocolates out of the blue. I get upset, and I don't understand why they can't support my weight loss efforts. It seems as if they are enabling my failure.

However, when I get my eating habits under control and people start noticing my weight loss, they usually compliment me. I am pleased, and it keeps me motivated. As I keep going, I end up losing a significant amount of weight. People suddenly look at me in a different way. I have felt invisible all my life, and all of a sudden I receive attention I don't know how to deal with. I feel like I am taken out of the bleachers and thrown into the arena. I become competition for people of my same sex and a subject of interest for people of the opposite sex. But I don't know the rules, and I don't know how to play. I feel attacked and preyed on, and I am scared.

I am so scared to finally be seen for who and what I am, to tell everyone when they hurt me or drive me to anger, to stop hiding in the shadow of my big body, and to present myself to the world. What if I am rejected or laughed at again? What if I am still not enough? What if there is still nobody who wants me? As long as I am overweight, I can blame all of these circumstances on my extra fat. But if I finally physically fit into social standards, and I still do not "fit in," then what? Then it means I really am worthless. Not because I am fat, but because I am me.

Fear drives my unconscious desire not to lose weight. Part of me cannot handle the idea of losing control of my reality as it is today and does not want to change, even if I don't like where I am. Today, being an overweight emotional eater is not exactly fun, but at least I know I can deal with it. I know the rules, and I know how to play my part. I feel in control over what happens to me. What if my weight loss brings me into a reality I cannot manage? What do I do then?

I can choose the disappointment of remaining an emotional eater forever, quietly hiding behind my walls of fat and playing a game I have mastered. Or I can choose the fear and anxiety brought by change, exposing myself to everything I have avoided until now, having no clue about really what to do and learning as I go. So far, I have chosen the security of silently eating my emotions. I don't know if I truly matter to my close friends and family. Why would it be worth the effort if, in the end, I still feel like I don't belong with those I love? I would rather give them a good reason not to love me and keep my extra pounds. At least I can blame it on laziness and lack of will, and I can decide that I am not good enough to be loved. It is easier this way.

Today, I have reached the point where I have more to lose if I don't change than if I do. I am tired of living a life full of disappointments, regrets, and unfulfilled expectations.

The Challenge: Self-Sabotage

Sabotage, from the French word *saboter,* means to destroy or to stop. When it comes to weight loss, the *sabotage syndrome* is any deliberate or unconscious thought, feeling, or behavior that attempts to destroy our ability to achieve our weight loss goals.

There are two common forms of sabotage in weight loss: self-sabotage and assisted sabotage.

- Self-sabotage is any behavior, thought, emotion, or action that holds us back from getting what we consciously want. It is the conflict that exists between our conscious desire to lose weight and our unconscious want to resist change that manifests in self-limiting patterns of behavior.

- Assisted sabotage happens when we unconsciously create or allow the sabotaging circumstances in our life and let others deliberately destroy, damage, or obstruct our weight loss efforts.

Sabotaging ourselves not only prevents us from reaching our goals, but also plays the part of a safety mechanism that protects us against disappointment. Our brain protects us from getting hurt by doing what it thinks is best, which is to keep us within the confines of our comfort zone.

Sabotage happens when we destroy our own ability to achieve our weight loss goals by working toward those goals and then retreating from them. Our own mind becomes our biggest enemy, and our thoughts begin to severely affect our behaviors. Sabotage is this ambivalent and harmful attitude toward ourselves that causes us to unconsciously do everything in our power to destroy our new, healthy lifestyle and keep eating our emotions.

Why We Self-Sabotage

Self-sabotage behaviors tend to appear because of a lack of self-esteem, self-worth, self-confidence, and self-belief. Negative thoughts about ourselves and our ability to lose weight can undermine our weight loss efforts. The messages we give ourselves through our conscious or unconscious self-talk have a powerful ability to affect our feelings, behaviors, and results.

Emotional eating in itself involves self-sabotage patterns. When we experience difficulty managing our daily emotional experiences, we tend to react to events, circumstances, and people in ways that obstruct our official desire to eat healthy. We rely on food to cope with stress, anger, sadness, boredom, loneliness, and other negative emotions rather than expressing them. As long as we need to eat our emotions, we will give ourselves good reasons to keep doing so and not control our eating choices.

Here are a few situations when we may use self-sabotage.

Coping technique. Self-sabotage is used as an effective method for coping with stressful situations or high expectations. We sabotage ourselves when we feel unable to reach expectations, set for us by others as well as self-imposed.

Combating fear—conscious or unconscious—of being deprived. For example, when I host a party and serve ice cream and cake, I really want to stick to my meal plan, but watching everyone else eat the goodies makes me feel left out and deprived. So either I indulge with my guests, or I wait for them to leave and then sneak into the kitchen and binge on what is left of the cake and the ice cream.

Fear of failure. When our previous attempts to get our emotional eating under control have failed, we see those failures as the worst thing in the world or as evidence of how inadequate we (consciously or subconsciously) believe we are. We choose never to really try again or self-sabotage our next attempts so we don't risk failing again.

Punishment. Some of us may also self-sabotage as a punishment. We believe we don't *deserve* to lose weight and be successful. So whenever we feel too close to accomplishing our goals, we destroy our progress and make sure to prove our negative beliefs.

Self-sabotage becomes our go-to technique for coping with challenging situations, the hassles of daily life, major life events, or unrealistic expectations of ourselves, which we subconsciously feel incapable of reaching.

Manifestations of Self-Sabotage

Here are a few signs that we may be actively self-sabotaging.

- We fear failure and we fear facing judgment when we don't meet our weight goals.

- We hold ourselves back from taking risks or changing our daily routines.

- We do not proactively change our diet because we fear we will make mistakes.

- We do not plan our meals ahead of time.

- We are incapable of saying no to others when they want to give us food.

- We don't take time to consider the consequences of our eating choices.

- We have too much pride to admit to our mistakes in our previous weight loss attempts.

- We set unrealistic expectations for ourselves, including unrealistic weight goals.

- We measure our own value based on what others do and eat and how easily they can exercise.

- We complain about people, life, unfair circumstances, or bad luck.

- We blindly accept other people's advice about nutrition and exercise.

- We regularly focus on what is not working or on wishful daydreams about what might have been or who we could have been.

- We compare ourselves with others, as in how much weight they have lost and what size of clothes they wear now.

- We compare ourselves to our previous selves when we were slimmer and in better shape and able to exercise harder.

How to Stop Sabotaging Your Eating Choices

Self-sabotage doesn't make sense. We make plans to start a new, healthy lifestyle, but we don't take action. We procrastinate, become self-critical, and make excuses. We engage in behaviors that seem to help in the short run, only to discover they are harmful in the long run.

We stand in our own way. Self-sabotage pushes us away from our deepest wants and desires. However, it's up to us to make the decision that we will no longer fall prey to our self-sabotaging patterns ever again.

Here is how to do it.

 ## *Identify Your Self-Sabotaging Behaviors*

You do not consciously try to destroy your efforts to eat healthier and lose weight. You do not carelessly play with your health on purpose. When a situation pushes you to eat, you are not at fault; you just automatically eat your emotions because this is what you have always done, and it has always worked. Eating helps you deal with some situations you may not know how to solve in a satisfying way.

Here are some of my own typical self-sabotaging behaviors and patterns of thought. Please check those that you use, too, and add any that impact you and are not listed.

☐ **"I lost three pounds, BUT I still have ninety-seven to go."**
I focus only on the negative aspects of my situation, ignore the positive, and cultivate a negative-thinker mindset. I actively discourage myself from putting forth more effort.

☐ **"I am going to fail."**
I hesitate or feel fear when I think about changing my way of eating. My fear of failure controls my thoughts and behaviors. I think that I will fail; therefore, I fail.

☐ **"If nobody knows that I cheat, it does not count."**
I eat in secret, feeling the need to hide from others. I build up my guilt every time, which pushes me to eat more to not feel it, and I am feeding the cycle of emotional eating.

☐ **"I am fat, ugly, not good enough."**
I have judgmental, negative, discouraging, and self-defeating thoughts. I beat myself up, and I am my worst critic. I cannot maintain my efforts when I don't feel worthy enough to change.

☐ **"I have to eat perfectly; otherwise, it means I have failed, so I might as well eat whatever I want for the rest of the day."**
I look for perfection all the time. If I eat a mouthful of cake, or if I don't end up looking like the Instagram models, it is not worth changing my relationship with food. I expect perfection for myself, adopt the saint-or-sinner mindset, and quit making an effort as soon as I fall for a spoonful of sugar in my coffee.

☐ **"I have never been able to lose weight and keep it off, so I won't be able to do it this time."**
I focus on my past failures and induce self-defeating behaviors to prove I am right to believe that I can only fail. I complain, but I don't really try to change anymore.

☐ *"I have so much weight to lose, I am never going to be able to do it."*

I jump to conclusions and make assumptions about what I can or cannot do. I focus on my final weight goal and freak out because it seems impossible, and it feels like the sky is falling on me. It is more than I can do, so I don't even try.

☐ *"It's too hard!" "It is my birthday, so I must have cake,"*
"My aunt made it, so I have to eat it," or "I have a slow metabolism."

I procrastinate and make excuses for not eating healthy or exercising. I am so good at it that I am not even aware these are excuses anymore. I truly believe what I say.

☐ *"I'm too tired, busy, or stressed out today,*
so I need to eat something good."

I accept my emotional eating as something I cannot overcome, and the ultimate solution when I am really upset and want to calm down.

☐ *"I will start tomorrow."*

I have the best intentions every night when my stomach is full and I feel ashamed, but the next day I forget how bad I felt the night before, and I repeat the same scenario over and over again.

☐ *"I know who I am as an overweight person,*
but I don't know who I will be when I am not, and it scares me."

My extra weight has become a part of my identity.

____

____

____

→ **Please take a moment to consider these behaviors. Which one (or more) do you think you use the most often?**

____

____

→ **In which situation(s) do you tend to use these behaviors?**

____

____

Congratulations! It takes a lot of honesty and courage to analyze your own self-defeating behaviors. This very important step will help you to create new, positive behaviors and take you closer to a healthier relationship with food. Good job!

Identify Your Sabotaging Triggers

Emotional triggers are those super-reactive places inside us that become activated by someone else's behaviors or comments. When triggered, we feel hurt or angry and withdraw emotionally. We tend to stay quiet and hide how we truly feel when these incidents happen, but we usually stay activated until we can release how we feel by eating. Because our feelings get so intense and painful, we need to eat them to defend against them. Our emotional triggers are wounds that need to heal. They are based on our fears. Being frequently triggered is exhausting and painful, and we use food to cope.

The way we deal with our emotions is the model we use to eat. It shapes our relationship with food.

As emotional eaters, our emotions are the primary cause of our eating behavior. There is a connection between the emotions you feel and your decision to eat. When you can identify the internal and external factors that trigger your emotions, you get a chance to modify your response to them. What is the signal that tells you, "Go eat now"? To what immediate stimulus do you respond?

In the coming days, please pay attention to the moments when you eat. Notice when you are not hungry and the situation you are currently in at the time, or the one you were in a few hours before you felt the urge to eat. Please try to keep this specific observation going until you can identify about ten triggering situations; the more examples you collect, the more you will be able to identify repetitive patterns. After a few days, analyze every specific situation, and try to identify exactly what triggered your impulse to eat. Your triggers may include people, objects, specific times, events, locations, emotions, thoughts, something you are told, or the way you are looked at. (I've provided a few examples on page 61.)

Please keep in mind that there is no need to blame yourself for what or how you eat as you put yourself under close observation for this exercise. Also, the point is not to try to resist your triggers at this stage. Our goal here is simply to identify, become aware of, and understand our self-sabotaging mechanisms.

◎ CONTEXT

I am having lunch with a few coworkers, and I catch one of them visually evaluating what is on my plate. I am upset all afternoon, and I get myself a huge dinner on the way home that I eat while expressing what I think of the coworker.

☀ TRIGGER

I can tell that this person was judging me. I feel disrespected, and it makes me mad. I should have said something and defended myself.

◎ CONTEXT

A family member tells me that I don't have the appropriate body shape to wear my outfit. I get upset and eat sugary treats all day long.

☀ TRIGGER

I doubt myself and feel inferior. I decide to wear something else that I can hide under.

◎ CONTEXT

____

____

____

☀ TRIGGER

____

____

____

◎ CONTEXT

____

____

____

☀ TRIGGER

____

____

____

➜ **Can you identify some situations that are similar or close? If yes, what is their common thread?**

____

____

➜ **Can you identify some triggers for your emotional eating? If yes, which ones are they?**

____

____

Identifying your triggers and what creates them takes a lot of self-awareness. You don't have to know all the answers right now; you can repeat this exercise as often as necessary. Please take the time you need to complete this exercise. Sometimes just keeping this in the back of your mind will allow you to become more aware of what triggers you to eat in the coming few days. You can also come back to this exercise each time you discover a new trigger over the coming months.

Neutralize Your Sabotaging Triggers

Our self-sabotaging behaviors are our automatic answers to our eating triggers. Once we have identified them, we can deactivate them and get some control back over our eating behaviors. When we become able to avoid giving an automatic answer to our triggers, we become more aware of what is happening, and we can then take conscious control of our thoughts, feelings, and actions.

To neutralize your emotional triggers to eat, you need to gently address the parts of yourself that feel flawed or about which you have self-doubt, such as your body image or your worthiness in all areas of your life. As you heal the initial wound and cancel your false belief, you set yourself emotionally free. Then you won't become as easily triggered the next time a similar situation occurs, and your urge to eat will become more and more manageable.

Examining the triggers you have identified on the previous page, please imagine one possible alternative reaction that would have made you feel better and neutralized your urge to eat. I've again provided examples to get you started.

✳ TRIGGER

During my lunch with coworkers, one person is evaluating what I eat and judging me. I feel disrespected, and it makes me mad. I should say something and defend myself.

◎ NEUTRALIZER

I allow myself to comment about what this person is doing at the moment it happens and let them know how it makes me feel. I am not upset all afternoon long and I don't need to overeat at night to compensate. I tell them something like, "I notice you are evaluating my plate. I feel judged. Please stop doing that."

✳ TRIGGER

When someone negatively comments about my outfit, I doubt myself and feel inferior. I decide to wear something else that I can hide under.

◎ NEUTRALIZER

I recognize my true worth and tell myself something like, "That's ridiculous. Of course that outfit fits me! No matter my body shape, I can wear whatever I want to."

✳ TRIGGER

◎ NEUTRALIZER

✳ TRIGGER

◎ NEUTRALIZER

Neutralizing your triggers is liberating because you don't get thrown off or drained by circumstances, your fears, or people's inappropriate comments or attitudes anymore. They may still be annoying, but they don't have the power to make you engage in sabotaging eating behaviors.

Jump-Start

→ On a sliding scale from 1 to 10, 1 for not at all and 10 for very much, how badly do you want to stop eating your emotions today?

1 2 3 4 5 6 7 8 9 10

→ On a sliding scale from 1 to 10, 1 for not at all and 10 for very much, how afraid are you that you will be left without "protection" if you were to lose all of your extra weight today?

1 2 3 4 5 6 7 8 9 10

→ What advantages does the part of you who does not want to lose weight see in staying overweight?

→ What fears come from the part of you that does not want to lose weight?

→ What is the worst thing that can happen if you stop eating your emotions and lose your extra weight?

➜ **If the worst thing were to happen, what are the ways you would overcome it?**

____

____

____

Thinking Outside the Box

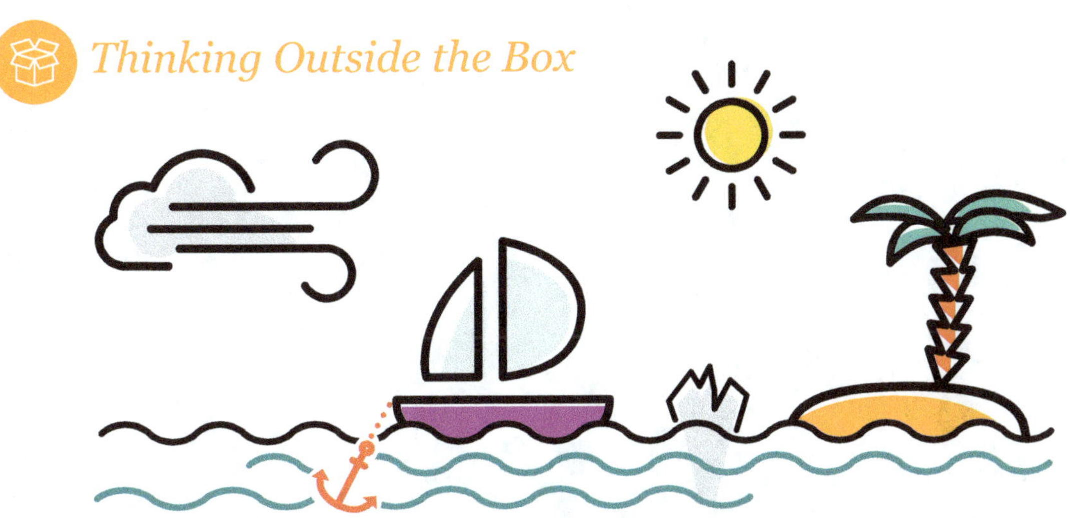

The goal of this coaching exercise is to help you envision your journey out of emotional eating. It will help you identify

- what can hold you back and the risks you have to take;

- your strengths and the resourceful behaviors you can use to increase your chances of success; and

- how to make your goals a reality.

Please take a stress-free thirty minutes when you will not be disturbed. Get comfortable, and imagine that you are on a boat sailing toward a beautiful, tropical island.

On the following page, please draw your own version of the artwork above. Begin by sketching a boat, sailing toward an island. Add an anchor, some reefs, the sun, some clouds, and the wind to your drawing. This is not meant to be a work of art, and it doesn't matter if drawing is not one of your top skills.

→ **After completing your sketch, please write your answers to the questions on page 67 near the corresponding element on your drawing to depict your journey to a healthier relationship with food.**

THE BOAT is the main element of the picture. It is a representation of you starting your journey to free yourself from emotional eating.

➔ **How do you feel as you get on board, leaving the past behind?**

THE ISLAND is a representation of your achieved goals at the end of your emotional eating recovery journey.

➔ **What are your goals as you cast off for your adventurous journey?** *(Consider new eating behaviors, activities, hobbies, mindset, lifestyle, or job; different types of relationships, traveling, type and size of clothing, body measurements, weight goals, etc.)*

THE WIND represents your strengths. In the same way the wind blows the boat's sails, your inner strengths allow you to move forward, reach the island, and achieve your goals.

➔ **What are your inner strengths that will fill your sails and keep you going, whatever happens, until you reach the island and accomplish your goals?** *(Such as a strong will, resilience, patience, persistence, ability to learn on the go, open-mindedness, ability to stay strong in adversity, positive mindset, and so on.)*

THE ANCHOR represents everything that holds you back and slows you down on your way to the island (internal factors such as fears, beliefs, emotions, feelings, body sensations, and attitudes).

➔ **What may hold you back and slow you down during your weight loss journey?**

THE REEFS represent obstacles and barriers that may appear on your way to the island and may threaten your goals (external factors such as environment, type of job, circumstances, and people).

➔ **What external factors may stand in your way as you sail toward the island and prevent you from accomplishing your goals?**

THE SUN is the help you can use while you are sailing that can make your journey smoother (such as people, emotional support, information, tools, and coaches).

➔ **What external help can you use to make your journey smoother and easier?**

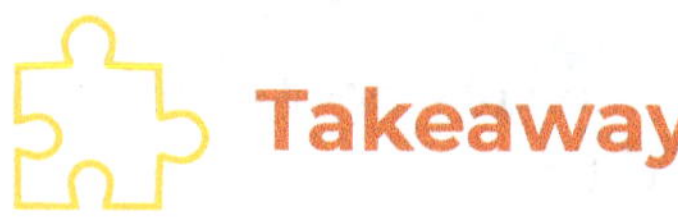

Takeaway

> *Self-destruction and self-sabotage are often just the start of the self-resurrection process."*
>
> —Oli Anderson

You are already successful!

Congratulations! You made it through this important step. It was tough, but you pushed through it. Every time you engage in negative self-talk, please remember you've come this far, and there is no way you could have done this without willpower or a strong desire to bring positive and long-lasting change to your life.

In addition, you are probably not a total stranger to what we discussed in this chapter. That means you have been on your way to recovery for some time. Let's capitalize on your existing achievements and experience.

➔ **What have you already tried/started/accomplished in the area discussed in this chapter that previously worked/was a success/was promising?**

____

____

➔ **What happened to get you started?**

____

____

➔ **What was your recipe for success?**

____

____

➔ **How can you use this proven successful recipe today?**

____

____

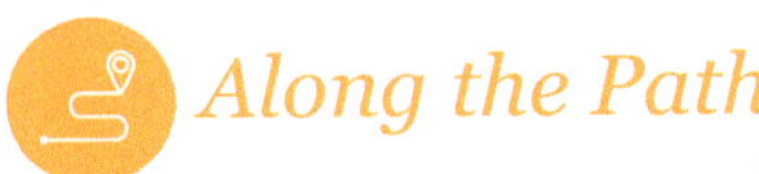 *Along the Path*

➜ **What have you been through while reading this chapter** *(what happened, how did you feel, what were your reactions, what important conversation did you have, did you have unusual dreams or body reactions/sensations)?*

____

____

➜ **What new perspective did you grasp in your relationship with food and with yourself or others or both?**

____

____

➜ **What new concept did you discover?**

____

____

➜ **What did you learn?**

____

____

➜ **What realization did you come to?**

____

____

____

➜ **What do you want to remember?**

____

____

____

Moving Forward

WHAT WILL YOU DO LESS?

✖

✖

✖

WHAT WILL YOU STOP DOING?

✖

✖

✖

WHAT WILL YOU START DOING?

✓

✓

✓

WHAT WILL YOU DO MORE OF?

✓

✓

✓

→ **Which one of these decisions will be the easiest for you to apply right now?**

You may feel what you have discovered and processed during this chapter is enough for you to successfully impact your relationship with food. This is great, and you are ready to jump into the next change. You may also feel it would be useful for you to dig deeper and explore these topics or some related areas a little bit more. If you want to take your reflection process and experimentation one step further, do this exercise.

WHAT ASPECTS DO YOU WANT TO EXPLORE MORE?

HOW WILL YOU MAKE THIS EXPLORATION POSSIBLE?

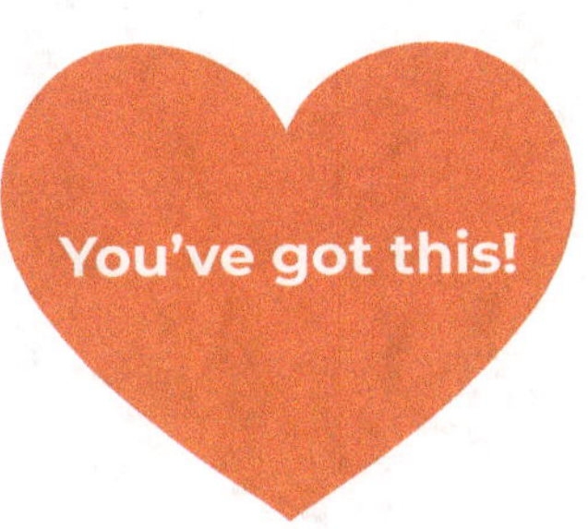

Develop Your Inner Balance

Your Inner Chaos Can Turn into Inner Peace

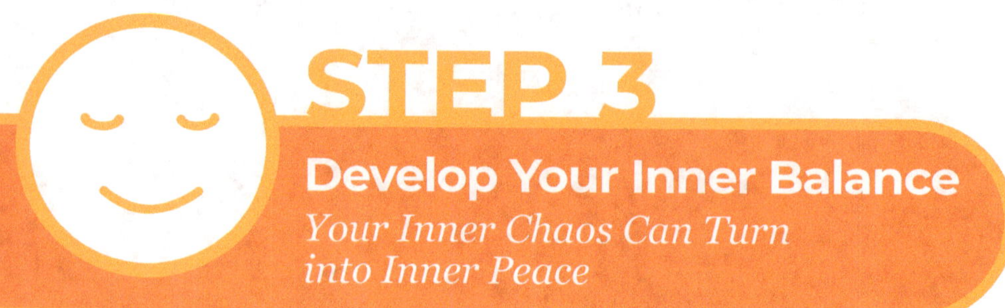

STEP 3

Develop Your Inner Balance
*Your Inner Chaos Can Turn
into Inner Peace*

I remember a day in second grade when my report card arrived and showed straight As. It was dinnertime, and my mother was about to serve my father first. As they discovered my grades, my mother was so proud that not only did she serve me first, but she also gave me what she was about to give my father: the biggest portion, with the best pieces of meat. I ate that dish like it was caviar. Being rewarded felt really, really good.

A few months later, another straight-As report card came in, but this time, nothing happened—no reward; it was just a regular day. I was very troubled, and when I went to bed that night, I could not sleep, trying to understand what I had done wrong. While my parents watched TV in the living room, I sneaked into the kitchen to get the reward I thought I deserved: I secretly ate a few treats. My father caught me. He punished me by humiliating me. He pulled me into the living room and then sat down next to my mother. I had to stand in front of them and repeat fifty times, "I am a fat cow who steals food, and I will always stay a fat cow." Then he sent me back to bed without a word.

Reward or punishment, whichever I would get, was not directly connected to me or my actions; it was connected to my parents' needs at that time and how facilitating or inconvenient I was to them. They were proud to have a smart daughter. My success was recognized, but not me. My success became their success in the same way my "bad behaviors" hurt their reputations and their sense of being good parents. How I felt or why I misbehaved was not the point. I was not a person in my relationship with them but "something" they had to deal with every day in their busy and stressed schedules that would make their day easier or create trouble for them.

They would reward me when I made things easy for them and punish me when I did not. I fully embraced that system, applying it to myself too. I wanted them to love me so badly that every "mistake" I made, greeted by the slightest annoyance I could observe in their reactions, would trigger self-punishing behaviors. The only thing I had access to at that time to fulfill the reward and punishment functions was food.

As an adult, eating is still my almost-exclusive way to show myself some signs of recognition in both a positive (reward) or negative (punishment) way.

Growing up, I was really confused by the difference between my behavior and action that would bring rewards my way and behavior and action that would make me feel good. They were often very different things. Sometimes I would feel awful and still be rewarded, and sometimes I was punished when I did not feel like I had done anything wrong. This distortion created a state of inner conflict that I have carried all my life.

What is good and what is bad? How do I know? If my inner compass cannot be trusted, what do I use as a reference? As a child, I used the way my parents felt and how they rewarded and punished me as a reference. As an adult, my compass is still the same: I focus on what pleases or displeases others to decide when I do good and when I do bad. I go for socialized norms, and I behave as it is expected of me, to make my environment feel good.

Most of the time, that means to shut up when I disagree, to not say a word when I feel angry, and to comply with demands even when I don't want to—all with enthusiasm, positive energy, and a big smile. At work, I follow a career path that does not give me a sense of fulfillment, but everybody tells me I would be crazy to quit. So I don't, and I eat at night to reward myself because I made it through another day, stuck in a cubicle living a meaningless life.

When it comes to dating, my attention is drawn to people who check all the boxes of "social attractiveness," even if we have nothing in common and even if they don't make me feel anything. When I feel awful after making an unethical decision at work, I reward myself with food because I was a good employee, doing what my boss expected of me. When I spend the weekend out with my friends but my mother rebukes me for not paying her enough attention, I stay with her the next weekend, giving her all my time and punishing myself with food for being so selfish and spending time away from her.

I don't do what feels right; I do what I get rewarded for. I don't ask for help, and I surely never take care of my needs. Eating is my maladaptive way to cope with my inner conflicts. Everything is mixed up, and I can never align what makes me feel good and what I have to do to be rewarded. I live in permanent inner chaos, and whatever I do, there is always a side of me that is not at peace. I don't know how peace feels. It is a state I am unable to reach. When I eat, at least I am able to reach silence. It is not peace, but it beats the raging storm.

Chaos is not mine. I was given it a long time ago, and I nurture it because I think I don't have the right to give it back. I am forcing myself into a life I think is the right one because I am expected to live it, but it is actually not the one that brings me peace. My current choices keep feeding my inner chaos. What if I switch priorities? What if I choose inner peace instead of a stable environment and meeting expectations? What if I trust my inner compass instead of what I get rewarded and punished for?

It is on me to choose with whom I surround myself and a life that fulfills me. It is on me not to silence my needs anymore. I can choose to let go of the expectations that were put on me. I can choose inner peace. When I don't adjust to what is expected of me, people who are disappointed leave me. It is hard to let them go. I feel guilty and rejected. But it allows me to meet people who are okay with who I am, what I do, and who I fit in with naturally, effortlessly. How I feel and what is expected of me finally align, and my inner storm begins to die.

When I am at peace, there is no more inner storm for food to calm. Eating my emotions as a coping mechanism becomes useless when there is nothing left to cope with.

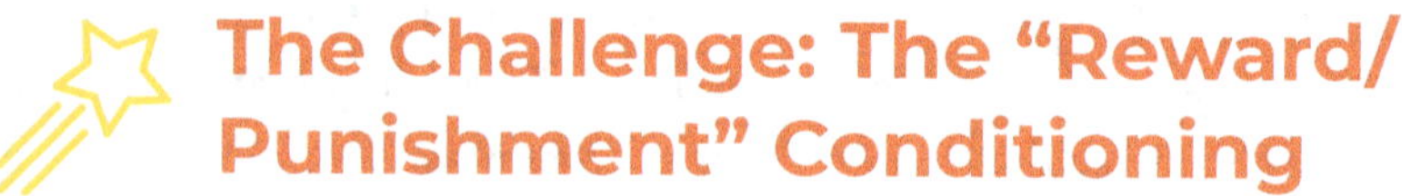 The Challenge: The "Reward/ Punishment" Conditioning

Operant conditioning is a way of learning by means of reward and punishment. This type of conditioning holds that a certain behavior and a consequence, either a reward or punishment, have a connection.

Punishment means a transgression. Reward means an obedience. Using this conditioning, we implicitly submit to a higher authority. We do not exercise our free will. We maintain ourselves in a state of dependency often seen as immature by others because it mimics the reactions of a child obeying their parents. We do not make the rules in our own life; we simply obey them.

Punishment and reward are always present at the other end of a demand, even a nonverbal or implicit one. When we make a demand to ourselves to meet expectations put on us, the only thing that matters is that we meet these expectations, whether it feels right or not, and no matter what it costs us emotionally. If we don't, we punish ourselves. If we do, we reward ourselves. Food as a reward or punishment is both the carrot and the stick for emotional eaters.

Consequences of Rewarding Ourselves

> *Rewarding is a process of increasing the frequency or rate of a behavior by means of presenting a stimulus shortly after the display of behavior. The stimulus that intensifies the likelihood of the behavior to be repeated is called a reinforcer."*
>
> —James Cangelosi

Reward systems are sometimes referred to as behavior modification. This is a system in which we are given a prize or bribe for certain desirable behaviors. Rewards are tangible items given to promote certain behaviors. For us emotional eaters, rewards will mostly consist of our favorite food. Yum.

There are two main issues with rewards.

1. While modifying the desirable behavior we want to display to satisfy a "higher authority," we may neglect our character development and not enforce our ability to make independent choices. This strategy implies that we do not know how to choose right from wrong if we don't get rewarded when we do good.

2. The reward system exists because we don't enjoy doing what we are demanded to do. It requires external motivation for us to comply with what is expected of us.

When we reward ourselves for activities or behaviors that are expected of us, we lose sight of the true value in an act that is right or wrong, good or bad, moral or immoral. Instead, we put our whole focus on the reward, which means that we are going to eat afterward.

As adults, we need to be able to value our actions in and of themselves. We need to choose actions for their intrinsic value so we are able to gain the confidence we need to succeed when we decide to stop eating our emotions. As long as we stay in reward conditioning, we feel insecure about our abilities to complete the required tasks to reach our goal on our own, and we seek a higher authority to guide us and confirm that we have done good. We blindly follow what we are told we need to do to break free from emotional eating and lose weight.

Consequences of Punishing Ourselves

In contrast to a reward, punishment is a process wherein a stimulus is presented after the display of an undesired behavior and causes the decline in the likelihood of the behavior. Education writer James Cangelosi writes that punishment is "a stimulus presented after a response to a demand, that decreases the probability of that response being repeated in the future." It is an easy solution to an undesirable situation in the short term.

But punishment comes with a detrimental, long-term side effect. When we know we face punishment, we are more likely to adapt our behavior to avoid the punishment rather than modify our behavior to what is acceptable. We do learn from punishment, but what we learn is how to avoid the punishment through lying and cheating behaviors (closet eating or not eating in public, for example). When our lies are exposed, the punishment becomes greater, and we become better at avoiding it. We enter the vicious cycle of eating on the sly.

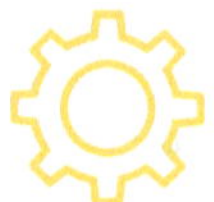

How to Heal the Core Wound of Humiliation

Beyond the obvious lack of freedom, the personal cost of reward-and-punishment conditioning is also the loss of connection and respect, both in terms of not being respected and of losing respect for the person having the power to make demands, who expects us to obey and who rewards or punishes us. We feel overpowered and humiliated. When we make demands on ourselves, we lose connection and respect for ourselves.

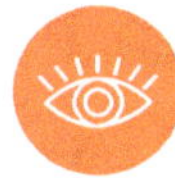 *Acknowledge Your Wound*

Humiliation is the act of feeling degraded, of degrading ourselves, or of excessively degrading someone else. This wound usually appears early in life. Parents may use shaming and humiliation to discipline their children. It happens, for example, when we are disciplined after experiencing something we enjoy, like eating. It can also happen in situations like getting dirty while playing, saying something inappropriate in public, being mocked by friends, being physically or sexually abused—multiple events can create a wound of humiliation.

Growing up, we feel shame when we perceive or believe we brought shame or embarrassment on our parents, authority figures, or the people we look up to, and our freedom is often impaired by their repressive attitude in response to what we did. We then start feeling durably devalued, ashamed, and humiliated.

Humiliation creates shame, self-criticism, self-blame, self-neglect, self-destructive behaviors, and the belief that we do not deserve for good things to happen to us. Here are the signs that I have felt, and you may feel as we suffer the wound of humiliation. Please check the ones that apply to you, and add those you feel but are not mentioned.

- ☐ I feel my body contains a lot of blocked energy, and I often experience tension in the neck, back, shoulders, throat, and jaw.

- ☐ I subconsciously seek pain and humiliation. Living with obesity is a perfect way to be judged and be given degrading looks and comments.

- ☐ I have difficulties expressing my needs and feelings because I fear I will be ashamed of myself.

- ☐ I show a lot of restraint in my words, control myself, and repress my impulses.

- ☐ I see myself as dirty, heartless, coarse, unworthy, and inferior to others.

- ☐ I tend to blame myself for everything and even take the blame for others.

- ☐ I punish myself before someone else does.

- ☐ I actually punish myself while believing I punish the other person.
- ☐ I understand my needs, but I don't listen to them because others come before me.
- ☐ I usually play "the parent role" in my relationships with others. I am their biggest fan, and our relationship is all about them. I take care of all their needs, but I don't express nor take care of my own needs in the relationship.
- ☐ I do all I can to be worthy in the eyes of the people I love.
- ☐ I take on a lot, which creates many constraints and obligations, thus ensuring that I am not free.
- ☐ What I do to free myself in one area imprisons me in another. For example, I want a good job that pays well so that I don't financially depend on anyone. But I hate my job, and I feel stuck having to spend every day there.
- ☐ Sense of duty is very important to me.
- ☐ I don't feel free to be myself in the presence of others.
- ☐ I cannot take in compliments from others, saying I just got lucky or I didn't really do all that much.
- ☐ I cannot take in positive expressions of love or admiration from others. I simply don't believe them.
- ☐ I pretend I don't care what other people think of me. I tell myself I am just fine the way I am. But in truth, I am hyperreceptive to any negative comment.

____

____

____

Freedom is important for me and usually to those who have suffered from humiliation. It is both our greatest fear and our greatest need. Here are the main fears that lead my own limiting behaviors and my resistance to access freedom. Please check the ones that apply to you, and add those that are not listed.

- ☐ I am convinced I cannot handle freedom; therefore, I subconsciously manage not to be free. Being overweight is an efficient way to limit my freedom in almost every area of my life.

- ☐ Being free for me means unlimited access to everything I like and having too much pleasure. I judge myself for seeking freedom, thinking, "This is not how one leads a decent life."
- ☐ I am scared of hurting others if I reveal my needs and desires.
- ☐ I am scared of being an egotist if I reveal my needs and desires.
- ☐ I am scared of being degraded or humiliated if I reveal my needs and desires.
- ☐ I feel unworthy to express my needs and desires.
- ☐ I don't even know what freedom really looks like, and feels like, for me.

→ **Which one of these fears and limiting behaviors do you display the most often?**

Great job! I know from experience that this exercise is tough and can rub on sensitive wounds that we would rather forget. It took me quite some time to admit all these affirmations applied to me. It may feel uncomfortable to explore the wound of humiliation, but remember, this is how you can stop letting it influence your life, choices, and mindset today. Please be gentle with yourself, and allow yourself to feel and express whatever emotions arise. They are all legitimate, and you are very brave.

 *Identify How You Cover Up Your Wound*

Humiliation victimizes us because it takes away our feeling of control over what happens to us. We are outraged, but there is nothing we can do to change the situation. When we think back about what happened, we believe we "should have" been able to defend ourselves, and because we weren't able to do so, we feel helpless and powerless, which causes us more humiliation.

We don't like to think of our humiliating experiences because they interfere with the image we have tried so hard to create of being competent, equal to others, and acceptable.

Here is what I typically do to avoid facing my own wound of humiliation.

- I convince myself that everything I do for others to "protect their feelings" is a great pleasure for me, including not saying anything when someone or something humiliates me.

- Whatever the circumstances and the pain I am truly in, I say everything is fine, and I try to have the biggest smile on my face.

- I find excuses for the people or situations that humiliate me.

We have to summon those difficult memories, though, because we need to discern the attitudes we use in order to stay away from what humiliation does to us. Coming to this realization is a difficult journey. It is not pleasant to admit we suffer from the wound of humiliation. Our ego usually does not make it easy for us and resists, creating several false beliefs to prevent us from being aware of our wound. Since many of our wounds are acquired in childhood, this is the time of our life we need to explore first, to get to the root of our wound of humiliation.

➔ **What are the most humiliating experiences of your childhood?**

____

____

Here are some of the excuses I find for the people who humiliated me so I don't have to face the truth of the pain those situations and relationships caused me. I cite my parents in the following examples because my core wound of humiliation first appeared in my relationship with them.

Please feel free to replace "my parents/my mother/my father" with the description of the person(s) or event(s) that originated your wound of humiliation. Please check the affirmations that match your own beliefs and attitudes toward them, and add those you use but are not listed.

- ☐ My parents were so young when I was born; they were just kids themselves and did not know what they were doing.

- ☐ My parents simply treated me the way they were raised themselves.

☐ My parents did their best; they had no clue they were hurting me.

☐ Life was so stressful for my parents at that time. They were on edge all the time. It is not their fault. They were great; circumstances simply pushed them into negative attitudes.

☐ My father has always been impulsive, and he would often regret his reactions afterward. You cannot change what you are and how you act.

☐ My mother thought the best way to deal with my father's anger was to avoid reacting in order to not make it worse. Her active attempt to protect me instead of staying passive may have made things even worse than they were.

____

____

When we suffer a wound of humiliation, our life is controlled by shame, and we tend to subconsciously reproduce difficult or humiliating situations in our own life as adults. This wound triggers a masochistic behavior pattern in us. As a consequence, a subtle and pernicious game plays out between our environment and us. Even if we are not aware of it, we feel like we can only exist and be seen and be recognized as weak and shameful—someone who is less important than others. Our environment tends to agree with us and treats us accordingly.

Here is how I feel and what I do when I am stuck in a masochistic behavior pattern. Please check the situations that apply to you, too, and add those that apply to you but are not mentioned.

☐ I criticize myself, laugh at myself, and devalue myself.

☐ I don't feel worthy of living a healthy life. I practice excessive and detrimental behaviors; excessive eating is just one of them.

☐ I feel unworthy of praise, compliments, and any kind of distinction.

☐ I subconsciously put myself in embarrassing situations.

☐ I tend to surround myself with people who do not respect me or who hurt me, or both.

☐ I do my best to earn others' love, and I do too much. I bend over backward to please others who appear to me to be fundamentally better than I am.

- ☐ I am always afraid of being a burden to someone else.
- ☐ I am always afraid of disturbing someone else or bothering them, so I try to be invisible and make myself as small as I can.
- ☐ I emphasize my sense of shame about my body by wearing clothes too small for me, that emphasize my fat rolls, do not totally cover my stomach, or let show my behind.
- ☐ I frequently stain my clothes with food or sauces.
- ☐ I choose to sit on chairs that are too small for me and are uncomfortable. I have broken a few chairs in public.
- ☐ I buy sweets in bulk and then feel ashamed at the checkout register.
- ☐ I disgust myself, and I find it legitimate that others are disgusted by me. I accept their disgust as the normal reaction to me.
- ☐ I neglect my physical appearance and create repulsion in others.
- ☐ I put myself into situations, although subconsciously, where I will be judged or compared to others, and where I will fall short of expectations.

We may find a subconscious satisfaction in experiencing humiliation. In my personal experience, when I am humiliated, at least I am seen. And being affected by obesity gives me a perfect opportunity to experience "easy" and frequent humiliation in a culture that values fit bodies.

Feeling humiliated leads us to eat our emotions. We eat to ease those difficult emotions we can't allow to come out. Admitting that we use a masochistic behavior pattern is not easy and highly uncomfortable, though. I personally grind my teeth with the simple evocation of the word *masochistic*. But when we manage to tell ourselves, "I use a masochistic behavior pattern, and this is why I react to some situations in ways that trigger my feeling of humiliation," the healing has started. When we can stop creating humiliating situations, we can stop eating the pain they create.

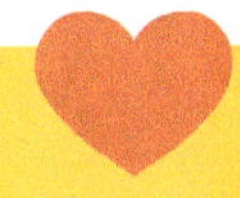

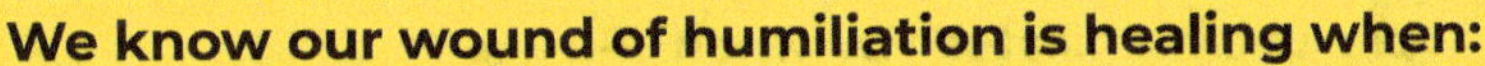
We know our wound of humiliation is healing when:

- we take time to check and fulfill our own needs before agreeing to others' requests;

- we take fewer responsibilities and feel freer; and

- we become able to make requests ourselves without feeling like we annoy others when we do so.

Let Go of Your Harmful Behavior Patterns

We have never been weak. We have simply done what we needed to do to survive. As long as we use our masochistic behavior pattern, we sincerely think it is the only way to protect ourselves, and in many ways, it is the truth.

Today, as adults, we have the ability to handle our wound of humiliation without engaging the protective behavior pattern that is now harming us more than helping us. We don't have to obey anybody else's demands. When we do, we choose to. We can stop surviving and start living. We are free.

Becoming aware of our masochistic behavior pattern is the starting point for letting it go. The more we feel the suffering the child in us has experienced, the more compassion we have for ourselves and the deeper we can heal.

➔ **On a sliding scale from 1 to 10, 1 for not at all and 10 for very much, how much have you suffered from humiliation as a child?**

1   2   3   4   5   6   7   8   9   10

➔ **On a scale from 1 to 10, 1 for not at all and 10 for very much, how aware are you today of using masochistic behavior patterns in your adult life?**

1   2   3   4   5   6   7   8   9   10

Allowing ourselves to have suffered and to have resented the people who originated our wound of humiliation is also necessary to let go of our hurtful pattern.

➜ **On a scale from 1 to 10, 1 for not at all and 10 for very much, how much have you resented the people who humiliated you when you were a child?**

1   2   3   4   5   6   7   8   9   10

➜ **On a scale from 1 to 10, 1 for not at all and 10 for very much, how much do you still resent today the people who humiliated you as a child?**

1   2   3   4   5   6   7   8   9   10

Please consider your most humiliating experience during childhood.

➜ **What do you wish someone had said to you right after that experience?**

____

____

Imagine someone you care about very much, someone you admire, is saying those words to you right now. Hear those words in your ears. Take those words into your heart. Notice how those words make you feel. Now, please say those words out loud to yourself. Take a deep breath and really take in those words.

➜ **How does hearing yourself say those words out loud make you feel?**

____

____

When we stop believing we still need to use masochistic behavior pattern to protect ourselves, we can become ourselves again. We can accept the fact that our wound of humiliation was one of the necessary experiences life has taught us to become who we are today.

No transformation is possible without acceptance. Acceptance is the trigger to start healing. Once we have become aware of our wound of humiliation, we can start accepting our masochistic behavior pattern and the fact that it was meant to help us when we created it. With this new attitude, we are able to see our wound of humiliation differently. We become able to tell ourselves that having used a masochistic behavior pattern to avoid suffering was a process of self-love because it helped us survive and adapt to our environment.

We don't need this behavior pattern anymore. We can stop creating the conditions to be humiliated. We can speak up when someone disrespects us instead of eating the way it makes us feel. We can let go of our extra weight and unhook the target we have hung on our backs.

As your wound of humiliation starts healing, you become able to check your own needs before saying yes to others' requests and expectations. You feel emotionally lighter, carrying a less heavy burden, and allow yourself more freedom. You become able to make requests without feeling like you are bothering others.

🔑 Jump-Start

→ **When was the last time you felt humiliated as an adult? What happened?**

→ **How did you react?**

→ **On a sliding scale from 1 to 10, 1 for not at all and 10 for totally, how satisfied are you with the way you reacted?**

1   2   3   4   5   6   7   8   9   10

→ **If you answered 5 or lower, how would you rather have reacted the last time you felt humiliated?**

➜ **What would you need to be able to react this way?**

____

____

➜ **When was the last time you felt inner peace and balance? What situation or context were you in?**

____

____

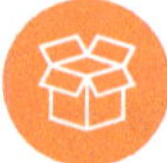

Imagine that you have a magic wand and can reach inner peace right now.

➜ **What is added to or removed from your life? How does it impact your behavior? Your relationships with others?**

____

____

Thinking Outside the Box

This exercise is adapted from _Presence_ by Amy Cuddy. It is designed to help you get back your sense of personal power. This body language exercise involves Amy's "power posing" because we don't just think with our minds, we also think with our bodies.

When we think of our body posture and facial expressions, we typically consider them to just be a display of what we are feeling inside. But Cuddy scientifically proves that our body language does not just communicate our thoughts and feelings to others; it also communicates our thoughts and feelings to ourselves. Our minds don't just influence our bodies; our bodies also influence our minds.

In this exercise, we will mimic very confident and dominant postures to temporarily boost our biology and psychology.

Amy Cuddy defined five main physical poses of high power.

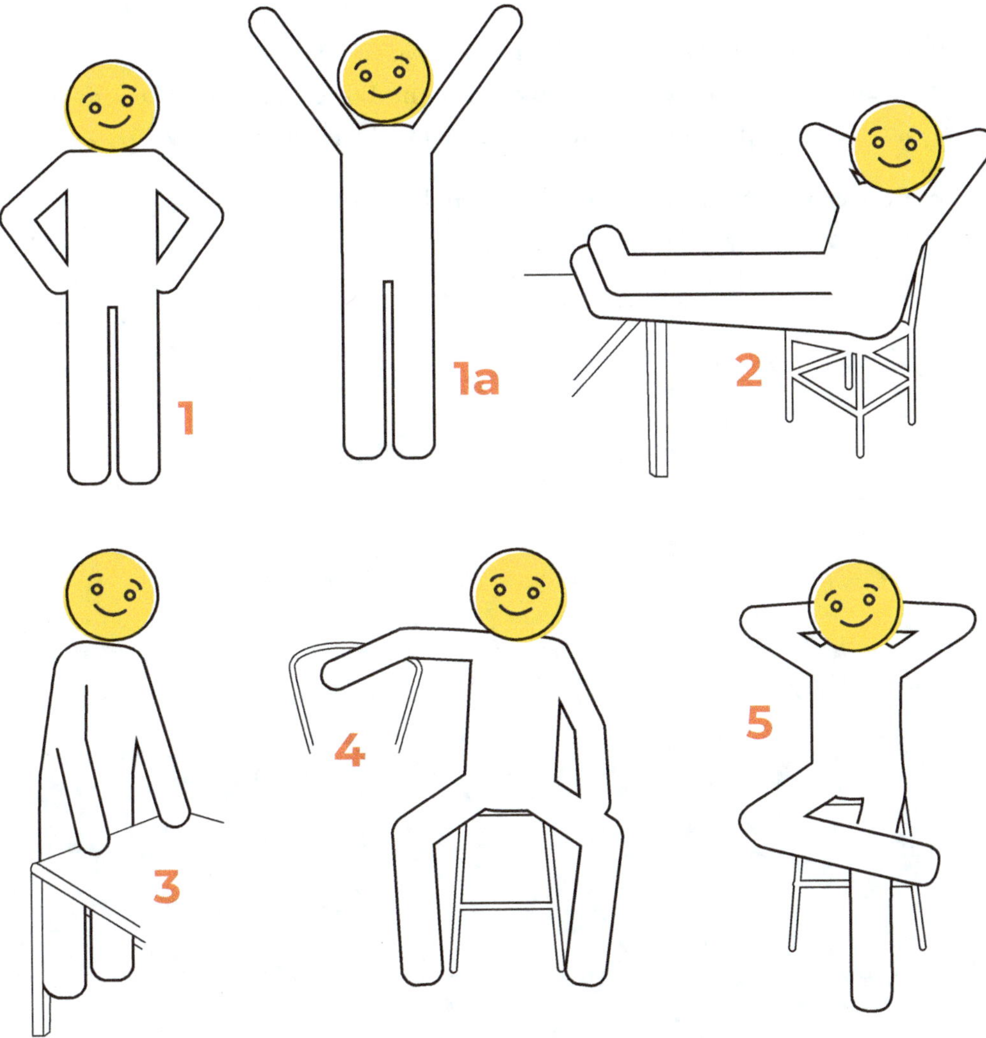

1. Standing, wide stance, puffed out chest, with hands on hips

1a. Variant: arms raised in a "V" above the head

2. Arms crossed behind the head, feet on table, leaning back

3. Hands planted on table, leaning forward, feet pointing straight ahead

4. Sitting, opening limbs extensively while keeping feet on the ground

5. Arms crossed behind the head, standing or sitting with ankle rested on knee

Please give yourself thirty minutes in a safe environment when you know you won't be disturbed and get comfortable. Pick the power pose you want to use today, and define a spot in the center of the room where you will power pose.

Choose three positive affirmations (for example: *I deserve to be respected. I am important. I am worthy of living a healthy life).*

Affirmation #1

Affirmation #2

Affirmation #3

Choose one of your favorite high-energy songs, turn on the music, and dance. You can replay the song or choose a medley of songs that you like. Dance until you can feel your energy has raised and you let the beat of the music guide your moves freely.

When you are ready, walk a few feet away from your power spot. Then walk toward your power spot with as much confidence as you can. Take your time, and stay tuned to your body sensations. When you arrive at the spot you have chosen, make your power pose, and hold it for two minutes. Two minutes is the minimum time necessary to impact our hormone levels. You can take longer, but if you hold the pose for less than two minutes, you will not get all the benefits from the exercise.

While you are holding your power pose, say your three affirmations in a loud voice. You may repeat them if you feel like it. If you feel like shouting them, just do. Take the time to clearly articulate each word. The point is not to fake it here but to really feel it. Please put as much intention as you can into your power pose and into your affirmations.

If you feel emotions, allow them to come out in whatever way feels right. You may also feel like slightly adjusting your power pose.

➜ **When you are done, please take a moment to evaluate your current emotional state and mindset. How are you feeling?**

____

____

____

If you wish, you can try experimenting in the future with other combinations of different power poses with different affirmations. Some may work together better than others.

If you like this exercise and how it makes you feel, you may turn it into a ritual; for example, every morning first thing when you get out of bed.

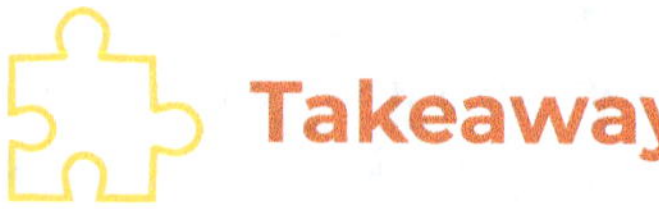

Takeaway

> *One's dignity may be assaulted, vandalized and cruelly mocked, but it can never be taken away, unless it is surrendered."*

—*Michael J. Fox*

You are already successful!

Congratulations! You made it through this important step. It was tough, but you pushed through it. Every time you engage in negative self-talk, please remember you've come this far, and there is no way you could have done this without willpower or a strong desire to bring positive and long-lasting change to your life.

In addition, you are probably not a total stranger to what we discussed in this chapter. That means you have been on your way to recovery for some time. Let's capitalize on your existing achievements and experience.

→ **What have you already tried/started/accomplished in the area discussed in this chapter that previously worked/was a success/was promising?**

→ **What happened to get you started?**

→ **What was your recipe for success?**

→ **How can you use this proven successful recipe today?**

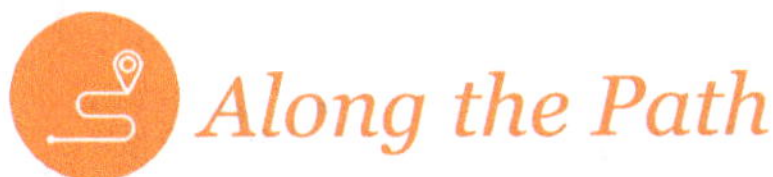

Along the Path

➜ **What have you been through while reading this chapter** *(what happened, how did you feel, what were your reactions, what important conversation did you have, did you have unusual dreams or body reactions/sensations)?*

➜ **What new perspective did you grasp in your relationship with food and with yourself or others or both?**

➜ **What new concept did you discover?**

➜ **What did you learn?**

➜ **What realization did you come to?**

➜ **What do you want to remember?**

Moving Forward

WHAT WILL YOU DO LESS?

✗

✗

✗

WHAT WILL YOU STOP DOING?

✗

✗

✗

WHAT WILL YOU START DOING?

✓

✓

✓

WHAT WILL YOU DO MORE OF?

✓

✓

✓

→ **Which one of these decisions will be the easiest for you to apply right now?**

You may feel what you have discovered and processed during this chapter is enough for you to successfully impact your relationship with food. This is great, and you are ready to jump into the next change. You may also feel it would be useful for you to dig deeper and explore these topics or some related areas a little bit more. If you want to take your reflection process and experimentation one step further, do this exercise.

WHAT ASPECTS DO YOU WANT TO EXPLORE MORE?

HOW WILL YOU MAKE THIS EXPLORATION POSSIBLE?

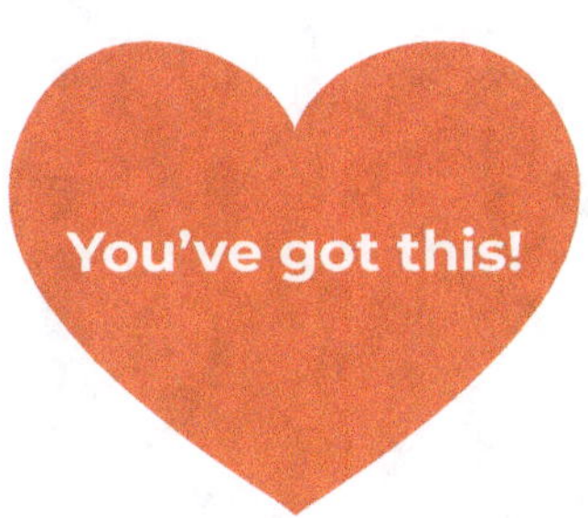

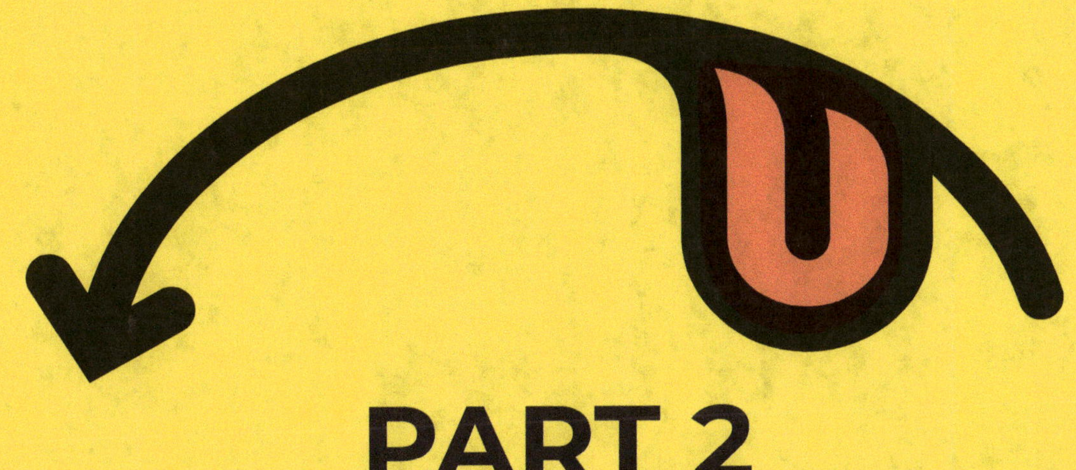

PART 2

From Emotional Compensation
to Emotional Release

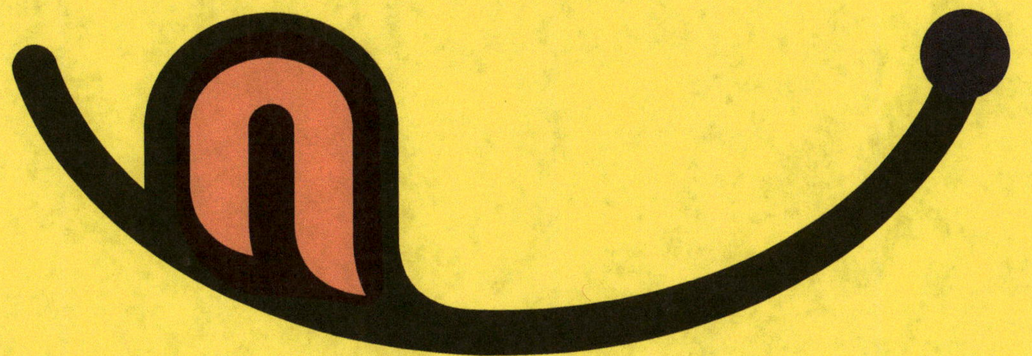

Connect Your Feelings to Heal the Pain

You Have Every Right to Feel the Way You Feel

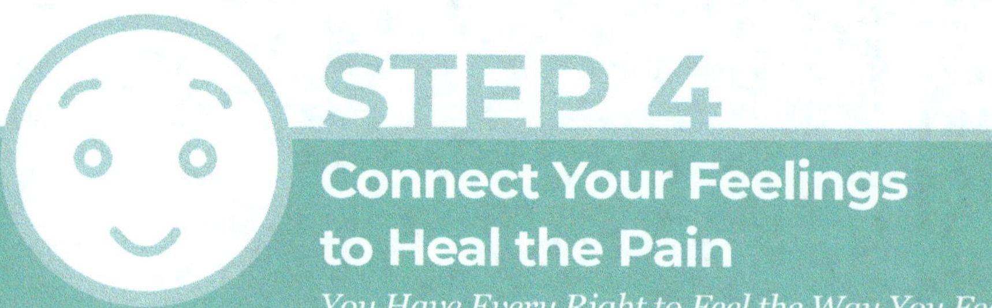

Connect Your Feelings to Heal the Pain

You Have Every Right to Feel the Way You Feel

I don't want to feel. It is too painful. I want to enjoy fun moments with my friends and family, maybe even experience slight disappointment sometimes. But I don't want to feel when my hopes get crushed, when I am rejected, when I feel useless, and when I blame myself for being humiliated, for not being heard or seen.

I choose to sacrifice happy feelings in order to stop being hurt so badly. I would rather not feel anything at all. I become absent from myself. I am physically here. I laugh at others' jokes, and I can even be the life of a party, but I make myself emotionally out of reach. I experience a great interior void that I try to fill with food. I am withdrawn from my own life, and boredom is never very far, so I escape boredom by snacking. When I am busy eating, I am not bored.

As years go by, my inner void and my emotional isolation grow, as do the boredom and the pain I need to numb. Not reflecting on myself, my life, and the choices I have made or avoided making has become vital in order to keep going. My abandoned self is now buried alive inside me. With the years, I have added a significant number of new wounds to the pain. It has become impossible to bring everything up in full light; it is best to simply keep eating.

When I eat my feelings, I use food to manipulate my emotions. I love what food does for me. I love the "feel good" feeling I get from a meal. I love the temporary fantasy that everything will be okay, if I can just get home after a bad day and crawl onto my couch with a bag of my favorite treats. I fill my stomach, but what is empty is actually not my stomach; it is my soul.

Overfeeding my stomach and living with my extra pounds is unpleasant, but the pain I would have to face to create a real connection with my soul terrifies me. I do not overeat because I am hungry or a glutton, or for the love of food. I eat my emotions because something painful is inside me, and I need to eat until I stop feeling it. I need to eat to distract myself from a pain I don't trust myself to face.

I choose to escape my pain with food because I can't escape the cause of my pain.

Food is my painkiller. It numbs me. Eating is an efficient way to avoid difficult emotions and not to hurt. But as I eat my feelings, I also cut myself out of the world. As I disconnect myself from the pain by eating, I also give away my joy, my sense of purpose, and my ability to trust myself and create meaningful relationships. I give up on myself. I burn all the bridges between me and my wounded self. I abandon the part of myself that cries in pain, and I am ready to let it die if that's what it takes to keep it quiet.

When I try to lose weight, and stop eating my emotions, my wounded self awakens quickly, screaming with pain. I am overwhelmed and unable to maintain the appearance that "I am fine, everything is fine," which I have been maintaining for so long thanks to food. I simply start to collapse. I have reached the point where I can't live my life if I am not numbed. I do want to lose weight, but not as much as I want to stay numbed. So I go back to eating my emotions and choose the lesser of two evils.

I am scared when I start digging into my emotions. I will have to make some unpleasant choices, create conflict with people I love, and cut some relationships with people I don't want to live without. I feel safer behind a calm and reasonable veneer, pretending I am fine and not creating trouble for the people I love. Whatever happens, and no matter how it makes me feel, I wield the shield of indifference and pretend it does not affect me, keeping everyone from seeing the crying and trembling me beneath.

As long as I need to numb my emotions, I cannot change my eating behaviors. Numbing my pain by eating my emotions, I hold onto my pain and never let it go. The only way out of my pain is through it, even if I believe that I cannot rise to the challenge. If I keep avoiding my pain, my eating habits will kill me anyway, with a heart attack or a stroke. Emotional pain cannot kill me, but numbing it with food can.

To die or to heal. Today, being affected by severe obesity puts me in a situation where not making a decision is actually making one. My extra weight is primarily a physical consequence of an unexpressed, unhealed emotional pain. I live with obesity because eating is the way I have found to not feel my emotional pain.

As long as I focus on the symptom (my extra pounds), and not on the cause (my emotional pain), I am stuck.

I want to lose weight, but I need to eat to numb my emotional pain. Logically, the less I want to listen to my pain, the more intense it gets, the more I need to eat, and the larger I get. How long do I want to silence my pain instead of dealing with it? How big can I get before pain literally kills me?

When I listen to my feelings rather than try to banish them, they provide information—clues that something may be wrong in the story I tell myself and the life I choose to live. My feelings are not my enemies. My pain has a meaning. It can serve a purpose. It can serve me instead of killing me. I am never wrong to feel. If I am in pain, it means something hurt me. I do not choose what hurts me or not, and I am never wrong when I get hurt. It is just a sign that something hurtful happened.

I eat my emotions when I judge myself or when someone tells me I *should not* feel hurt. I think I don't have the right to be hurt, so I don't express my feelings when I am. I repress the pain and numb myself with food. When I allow myself to fully experience painful or uncomfortable feelings, I work toward my healing. I can let go of the guilt of not trying hard enough to be happy with what I have. I can stop believing that every time I hurt, it means I am the one doing something wrong. Every moment I accept to feel the pain, I heal. Painful emotions are impermanent. They just need a way out. They simply need my permission to exist, follow their course, and then leave me.

The Challenge: Emotional Invalidation

Emotional invalidation occurs when our emotional experiences, feelings, or thoughts are rejected, ignored, or judged. Invalidation disrupts relationships and creates emotional distance between us and others as we repress the way we feel.

We are often unaware of how we invalidate ourselves and how numbing ourselves with food also disrupts our relationship with ourselves, creating an emotional distance between our sensitive self and our judgmental self.

We invalidate our feelings when we react to them as if they are not valid or reasonable. Validating our feelings doesn't mean we have to agree with them. It doesn't mean they are the healthiest or informed by logical emotional reactions. Validating our feelings doesn't make them more true. A validated feeling does not hurt more than a rejected one. Validating our feelings simply means we allow ourselves the right to feel things we don't always understand at the moment we feel them.

Invalidation can happen with painful feelings and also with positive feelings. When we have deep pain within us, sometimes we cannot allow ourselves to relax and enjoy our lives. We cannot just have fun because doing so would not feel right; it would feel offensive or even like a betrayal to somebody or to the past.

Validation is about accepting instead of judging ourselves. To validate our feelings is first to accept our feelings, then to understand them, and finally to nurture them. To validate is to acknowledge and accept who we are. Invalidation, on the other hand, is to reject, ignore, or judge what we are and what we feel.

Validating a feeling we agree with comes naturally. Validation is not as easy when we deal with feelings that we disagree or are in conflict with. It can be difficult to find something to validate in the way we feel while remaining true and loyal to what is expected from us and to the people we love. Even though we know that listening carefully to our feelings is important, it can be very difficult to recognize when we don't.

 ## What Happens to Our Invalidated Feelings?

Invalidated feelings don't just vanish. They stay with us, and they still run their course of action inside us. We are just not aware of their presence. We do not allow ourselves to feel them, so we try to get rid of our feelings, and we eat to dissociate ourselves from what we feel. Thanks to disassociation, we can keep our feelings out of awareness, locked up inside us like a part of the hidden "not me."

Consequences of Emotional Invalidation

The emotions we feel and the thoughts we think can have a direct impact on our physical health. "Studies have shown that chronic pain might not only be caused by physical injury but also by stress and emotional issues. . . . Often, physical pain functions to warn a person that there is still emotional work to be done," writes Dr. Susanne Babbel, a psychologist specializing in trauma and depression. Can we consider our extra weight as a physical pain function? Functioning with my own obesity does create physical pain for me (shortness of breath, joint pain, difficulty sleeping), so I would say yes.

In our relationships, when we cannot validate our own feelings, we go on a never-ending quest to try to make others do it for us. Whatever maladaptive coping mechanisms we use, it never works, and we never really get what we need. We don't heal the past, and we hurt our present relationships.

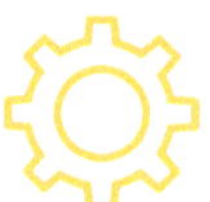

How to Connect with Your Feelings

Life is full of emotional distress, and emotional stress can be quite challenging. By definition, we emotional eaters do not have a healthy relationship with our emotions. More often than not, we choose to repress and eat the negative emotions we don't know how to relate to or handle. Instead of processing these emotions, most of us subconsciously learn to avoid them or push the discomfort away by eating them. We eat an "emotional pain" sandwich. Yummy.

We silence the pain and bottle up our fear, sadness, and anger. It comes at a high cost too. The more we hold something back or try to force it away, the stronger it becomes. The more emotions we repress, the more inner conflicts we experience and the more anxiety we feel as we keep our true self silent to maintain the illusion that we are fine.

Identify How You Detach from Your Emotions

Ignoring our feelings is an emotional abuse we inflict on ourselves. Emotional eating is a flat-out dismissal of our emotions. We are basically telling ourselves our feelings don't count, whether we don't agree with them or we are uncomfortable dealing with them. In the process, we may misunderstand, not pick up on, minimize, criticize, or even pathologize our feelings.

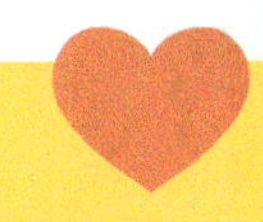

We don't ignore our emotions by eating them out of choice or because it feels good.

We learned to detach from them, using food, because at one point, we needed to disconnect from our feeling self in order to survive. The pain was too intense for us to process. As long as an emotion is not processed, it sticks with us, intact. Whatever we numbed with food is still with us; we just cannot feel it anymore.

It may be difficult to detect the moment when you reject your emotions. What occurs can be very subtle, but it leads to a quiet and slow erosion of your self-value. Through a simple thought like "Oh, grow up" or "You're asking for too much," you are rejecting the validity of what you feel. Eating these invalidated emotions comes right after.

Here are a few of the behaviors I use today when I reject my feelings. Please check those that apply to you, too, and add those you may display and are not listed.

- ☐ *I don't make a decision without asking for somebody else's opinion.*
  Example: I ask my close friends' opinions about strictly personal matters when I start dating somebody or when I think of switching to another job.

- ☐ *I reject my emotions as soon as they appear.*
  Example: When my partner does something that hurts me, I tell myself, "There's no way I can be mad at them right now. Not after they just took me out to dinner."

- ☐ *I let others tell me how I really feel.*
  Example: I feel humiliated by my partner's attitude, but they tell me, "You're just jealous because you think I was flirting with the waiter/ waitress." And I find myself agreeing with that affirmation.

- ☐ *I let others tell me how I should feel.*
  Example 1: My partner tells me, "You should be grateful that I care so much to pay for our rent and our groceries," and I feel guilty to have a negative emotion instead of showing gratitude.
  Example 2: During an argument, my partner tells me to "just relax," and I immediately control the tone of my voice and the speed of my speech, or I simply shut up.

☐ *I ignore my feelings; they are not important enough for me to address.*
Example: I really need a couple of days off. I am exhausted and need some quiet and alone time. My family wants to spend the weekend in an amusement park. I do not want to go but they all push for it, so I go anyway.

☐ *I think that what I feel is my fault.*
Example 1: When I get upset, I tell myself, "You are too sensitive." Doing so, I reject any unhappiness I feel at that moment. Then, since I am "not really unhappy, just being sensitive," there's no need to talk about why I am unhappy. And I swallow the whole thing down, usually with ice cream.\
Example 2: "If I could just learn some trust, I wouldn't feel insecure when my partner comes home at 3:00 a.m.," when coming home that late actually is a big red flag.

☐ *I am dismissive with myself. I tell myself why I don't want to feel mad, hurt, sad, or a certain way.*
Example 1: I get upset and I tell myself, "This is pointless. I am just overreacting."
Example 2: I am hurt because I did not get a birthday card from my family, but I think, "Who cares about getting a birthday card anyway?"

The reason for feeling an emotion is always valid. Whatever you feel, you are *right*. You cannot be wrong just because you feel something. You are always right to feel what you feel. Whatever happens, your emotional response is legitimate and valuable no matter what this response is, and even if people around you don't want to deal with your reaction.

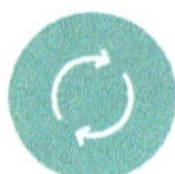 ## Disengage Your Survival-Mode Answer

When we suppress our emotions, we use an automatic defense mechanism. We switch to survival mode because we read our feelings as a potential threat. When we activate our survival mode, we disconnect the prefrontal, rational, thinking part of our brain and activate the reptilian, instinctive part. From there, only three possible behaviors exist: assault, freeze, or flight.

Emotional eating is a flight survival answer. We feel so threatened by our feelings that we automatically run away and disconnect. After a difficult day at work, for example, we know we are not going to die because we disagreed with our boss. Still, we feel the urge to eat.

This might sound a little extreme when it happens to us as adults. But if earlier in life we openly disagreed with an authority figure and their reaction deeply frightened us, then we learned that to openly disagree with a figure of authority can actually feel life-threatening. So now, every time we disagree with our boss at work, our survival mode is activated automatically. We simply shut up and eat our frustration away when we are alone and feel safe in our home.

There was a time when you expressed your emotions freely or witnessed someone doing so. Something then happened that taught you that you should not have. Now, you don't think twice, and you automatically repress most of what you feel by eating.

→ **Please think about what happened during one occasion when you freely and totally expressed anger, joy, sadness, fear, disgust, and surprise. You may have to go back several years, depending on how long you have suppressed these emotions.**

ANGER

Example: As a child, my father wanted me to do some chores after my homework when I was promised I could have some leisure time. I angrily refused. He forcibly confronted me and then forced me to deep-clean our house from attic to basement.

What Happened: ____

____

____

JOY

Example: I lost three pounds. I was excited and wanted to share my joy with my partner. When I did, they reminded me how much I still have to lose. All my joy was instantly gone.

What Happened: ____

____

____

SADNESS

Example: As a teenager, I just broke up with the first person I ever dated, and I needed some support from my mother. She told me that dating them was a bad decision, and she actually was happy we broke up. She told me she didn't want me to bother her with useless tears.

What Happened: _______________________________

____

____

FEAR

Example: As a child, my mother wanted me to do something that frightened me. When I told her I was scared, she got mad, shamed me, and called me a coward.

What Happened: _______________________________

____

____

DISGUST

Example: As a child, my father cooked meat for my dinner. It smelled bad, and I told my father it disgusted me. He got mad, told me that this was expensive meat, and forced me to eat it all. I was sick all night.

What Happened: _______________________________

____

____

SURPRISE

Example: As a child, I was alone dancing in the living room. When I turned around, I saw my parents looking at me. I was so surprised that I missed a step and almost fell. They laughed at me.

What Happened: _______________________________

____

____

➜ **Regarding these memories, please remember the conclusion you drew after those events happened:**

ANGER
Example: When I express my anger, things only get worse for me.

Conclusion Drawn: _______________________________________

____

____

JOY
Example: When I show my happiness, people steal it.

Conclusion Drawn: _______________________________________

____

____

SADNESS
Example: Others don't want to support me when I am sad. They reject me and hurt me more than I already am.

Conclusion Drawn: _______________________________________

____

____

FEAR
Example: Expressing my fear doesn't get me help and exposes me to disparaging judgment from others.

Conclusion Drawn: _______________________________________

____

____

DISGUST

Example: Expressing my disgust makes others mad at me. I would rather lie to avoid what disgusts me or endure it quietly to not make things worse.

Conclusion Drawn: _______________________________

____

____

SURPRISE

Example: I need to always stay in control and never get caught off guard or it will be used against me. I cannot allow myself to be vulnerable.

Conclusion Drawn: _______________________________

____

____

When our survival mode is activated today, we engage in emotional eating because we fear feeling an emotion we have learned to refuse. We therefore display defensive behaviors.

- We **ban** and suppress every feeling that makes us feel uncomfortable and every signal of discomfort that our body could send to alert us by eating.

- We **blame** ourselves for the consequences of our eating behaviors and our extra weight, creating guilt and a feeling of worthlessness.

- We **victimize** ourselves, believing we don't have control over our eating choices.

- We **justify** our reactions by giving external explanations for our eating behaviors.

You can disengage your survival-mode answers to your emotions when you learn to trust yourself to face your emotions. As your level of fear and refusal lowers, you can

- **observe** your body reactions and your sensations without judging them or blocking them;

- **investigate** and put words on what happens inside you, identifying what generates that emotion for you;

- **let go** of your urge not to feel discomfort and unpleasant emotions; and

- **move toward** yourself and embrace the way you feel.

Learning to trust your emotions, when you have learned to not trust them previously, is an act of faith in yourself. It is not easy, but you are worth it. You don't have to go from zero to a hundred in a split second. You can learn progressively and allow yourself baby steps when the situation feels safe enough for you to experiment with this new attitude.

 ## Develop Your Self-Awareness

We view negative emotions as something we should not have to experience, and we resist them. But repressed emotions can destroy our relationships and make us miserable. Eating our emotions leads us to obesity and threatens our lives, not to mention our happiness.

Communication is the key to a successful relationship between your feeling self and your judgmental self. When you shut down your ability to listen to what you feel, you turn your inner dialogue into a one-sided conversation where you can only hear your critical inner voice whispering negative statements and judging you when you overeat. You mute the part of yourself that tells you what you need and this triggers your urge to eat.

When you find yourself eating your emotions or about to eat them, you can pay attention to your inner voice. Which one is leading right now? Your feeling self or your judgmental self? How much are you really in tune with your feelings? How much are you evaluating what you feel? Are you analyzing, reasoning, and intellectually deciding you don't want to feel a certain emotion and trying to reach the emotion you think you should feel instead? How do you use food to reach the desired emotion and mute the one you actually feel?

Here are some markers that I use to identify my inner state when I eat or am about to eat. Please, during your next meal, define where you stand for each marker.

I don't smile   ⟶   I smile

1   2   3   4   5

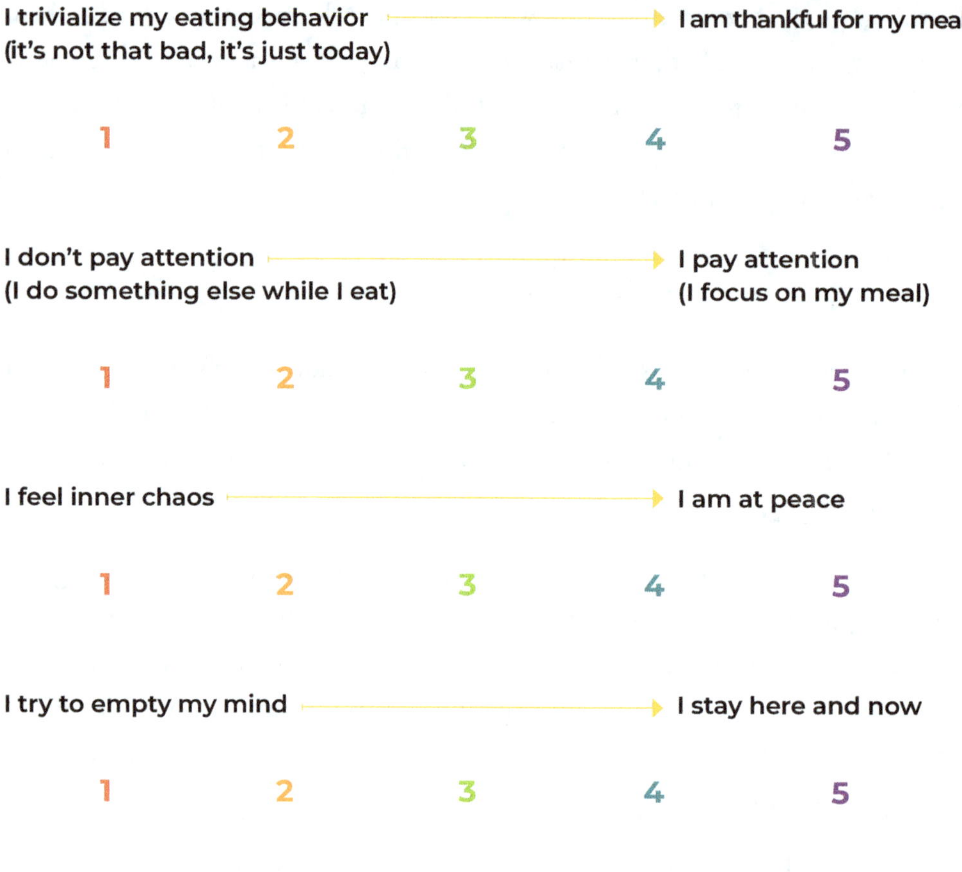

➔ **What is your total score?** _______ / 25

- The higher you score, the more you allow yourself to be in tune with what you really feel as you eat. If you score high, you probably are not eating your emotions during that meal but are simply feeding your body.

- The lower you score, the more your judgmental inner voice is in charge at the moment you eat. You are probably eating your emotions, methodically numbing yourself.

- If you find yourself not willing to do this exercise and simply avoiding it as you are eating (whatever excellent reason you may invoke), it is a strong sign, at that moment, that you are totally removed from your feelings, and your judgmental self is 100 percent in charge. You are definitely doing your best to suppress your feelings at this moment.

➔ **What does your score tell you?**

____

____

You can use these markers as often as you want to, right before or as you are eating, to help you detect how connected to your emotions you are during your meals.

Accepting an emotion does not mean that you agree with your feelings. You simply accept that you will get back in touch with your feelings without trying to talk yourself out of the feeling or shaming yourself for feeling this way. When you learn to accept your feelings, your emotions are no longer threats, but informants. They show you who you are, what you care about, and what matters to you. They serve you. You can then identify what triggered your emotion and what causes your eating response.

Emotions keep us attuned with who we are. What is the meaning of our lives if we cannot feel anything?

How can we find our purpose if we go through life being numb? When we accept emotions are a natural part of our experience, we can let them be. If we let them be, we don't need to eat them anymore.

🔑 Jump-Start

➔ **Remember one past event that hurt you. What happened?**

____

____

➔ **What did you feel (body sensations, feelings, and emotions) when it happened?**

____

____

➜ On a sliding scale from 1 to 10, 1 for not intense at all and 10 for extremely intense, how intense were your feelings when it happened?

1   2   3   4   5   6   7   8   9   10

➜ On a sliding scale from 1 to 10, 1 for 10 percent and 10 for 100 percent, to what extent did you express the intensity of what you were feeling?

1   2   3   4   5   6   7   8   9   10

➜ What did you actually express? What did you say and what did you do in reaction to that painful event?

____

____

____

____

➜ What would you really have liked to have done and said?

____

____

____

____

➜ What made you choose not to express your true feelings?

____

____

____

____

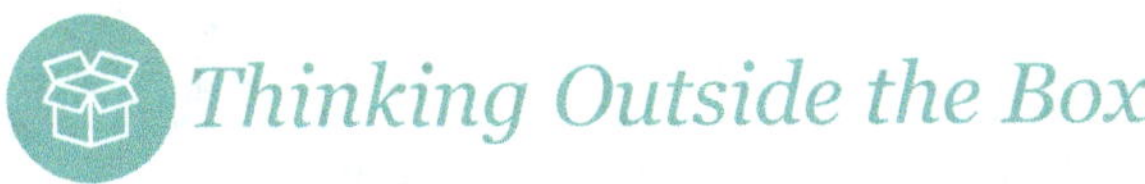 *Thinking Outside the Box*

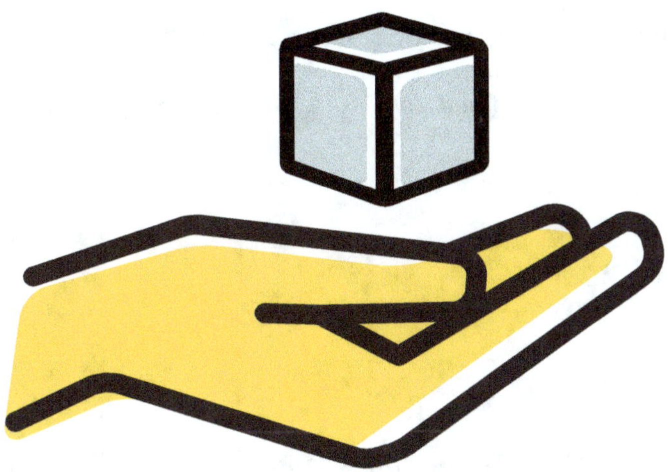

This body-mind exercise is designed to help you get back in touch with your sensations, feelings, and emotions.

Please give yourself twenty to thirty minutes at a time when you know you will not be disturbed. Take an ice cube in your hand and close your fingers around it. Pay attention to the first reaction that pops into your head. For example, it can be pain, the impulse to throw the ice cube away, the impulse to shout, muscles getting contracted, clenching your jaw, running around, or saying out loud, "This is cold!"

➔ **What is your immediate reaction in the first moments when you put the ice cube in your hand?**

Example: I throw it away after twenty seconds.

____

____

____

____

With the ice cube still (or back!) in your hand, force yourself to come to a standstill and to keep quiet for two minutes. Pay attention and welcome all your body sensations, emotions, and thoughts.

➜ **What does it take for you to stand still and be quiet?**

Example: I need to distract myself from what I feel by singing a song in my head.

____

____

____

➜ **What are your emotions? (Fear, anger, sadness, something else?)**

Example: I am irritated.

____

____

____

➜ **What are your body sensations? (Cold, humid, hot, stinging, something else?)**

Example: My hand is so cold that it starts stinging. It is unpleasant, and I start hurting.

____

____

____

➜ What body sensations can you feel in your face area and in your heart area?

Face Example: I am getting red, my cheeks are getting warm, and I am clenching my jaw.

Heart Example: I have a feeling of oppression in my chest and my heart beats faster, pounding hard.

➜ What thoughts are emerging right now?

Example: I do not like this exercise. Why on earth am I doing this? Why am I forcing myself into something so unpleasant?

The same process takes place when we replace the ice cube with an emotion that does not feel good: to express it is more natural and painless than to force ourselves to contain it while pretending nothing is happening.

Accepting what we feel and taking action according to what we feel with this exercise allows us to go beyond the repression of our emotions and acknowledge the messages our body sends us instead of numbing ourselves. We become aware that we spend a lot of energy controlling ourselves to be able to stand still as we experience sensations and emotions that we repress.

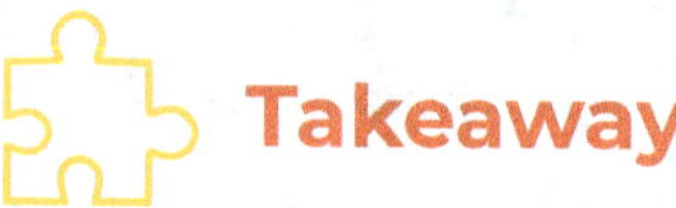

Takeaway

> " Let everything happen to you, beauty and terror, no feeling is final."

—*Rainer Maria Rilke*

You are already successful!

Congratulations! You made it through this important step. It was tough, but you pushed through it. Every time you engage in negative self-talk, please remember you've come this far, and there is no way you could have done this without willpower or a strong desire to bring positive and long-lasting change to your life.

In addition, you are probably not a total stranger to what we discussed in this chapter. That means you have been on your way to recovery for some time. Let's capitalize on your existing achievements and experience.

➜ **What have you already tried/started/accomplished in the area discussed in this chapter that previously worked/was a success/was promising?**

➜ **What happened to get you started?**

➜ **What was your recipe for success?**

➜ **How can you use this proven successful recipe today?**

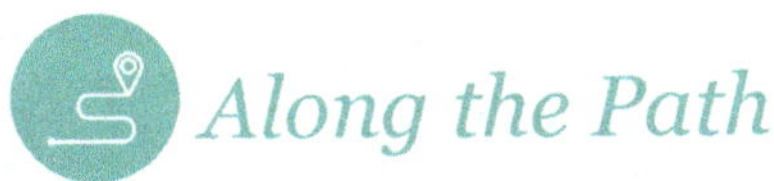

Along the Path

➜ **What have you been through while reading this chapter** *(what happened, how did you feel, what were your reactions, what important conversation did you have, did you have unusual dreams or body reactions/sensations)?*

➜ **What new perspective did you grasp in your relationship with food and with yourself or others or both?**

➜ **What new concept did you discover?**

➜ **What did you learn?**

➜ **What realization did you come to?**

➜ **What do you want to remember?**

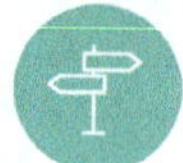 ## *Moving Forward*

WHAT WILL YOU DO LESS?

✖

✖

✖

WHAT WILL YOU STOP DOING?

✖

✖

✖

WHAT WILL YOU START DOING?

✓

✓

✓

WHAT WILL YOU DO MORE OF?

✓

✓

✓

➜ **Which one of these decisions will be the easiest for you to apply right now?**

You may feel what you have discovered and processed during this chapter is enough for you to successfully impact your relationship with food. This is great, and you are ready to jump into the next change. You may also feel it would be useful for you to dig deeper and explore these topics or some related areas a little bit more. If you want to take your reflection process and experimentation one step further, do this exercise.

<table>
<tr><td>WHAT ASPECTS DO YOU WANT TO EXPLORE MORE?</td><td>HOW WILL YOU MAKE THIS EXPLORATION POSSIBLE?</td></tr>
</table>

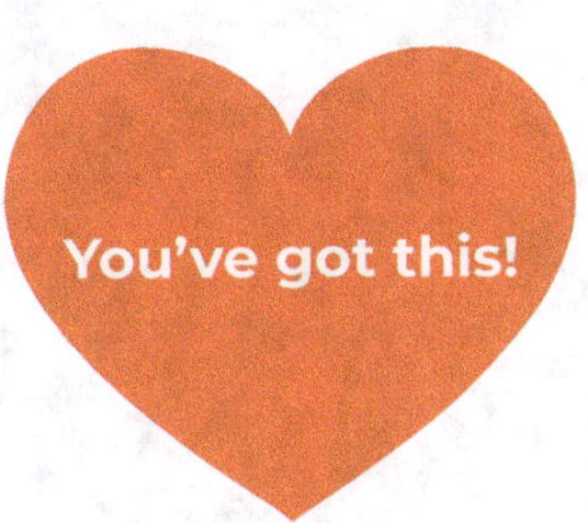

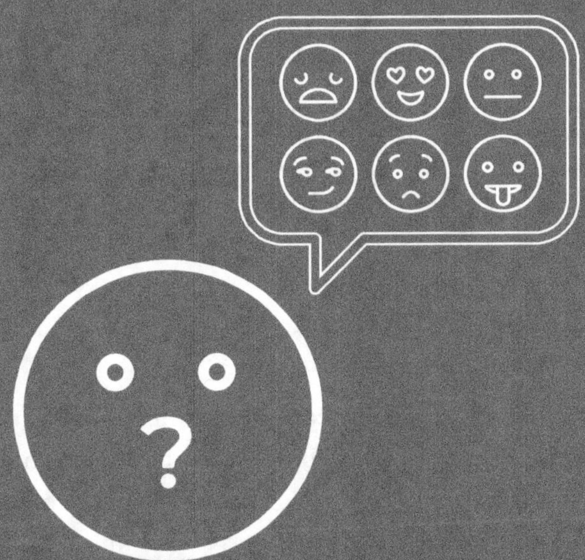

Name Your Emotions to Identify What You Need

How You Feel Tells You What You Need

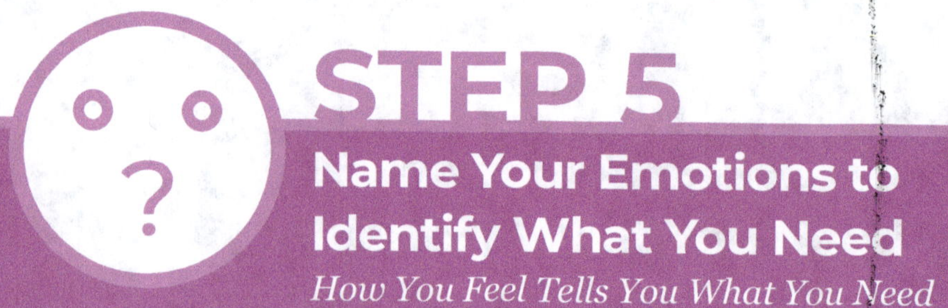

STEP 5

Name Your Emotions to Identify What You Need

How You Feel Tells You What You Need

"I'm fine."

Whether I am holding my tears or clenching my fists, this is the answer I give every time I am asked how I am doing. It has become so normal to me that when I am asked, "What are you feeling right now?" I am unable to answer. Most of the time, I don't know how I feel. I feel *something*. I know that my throat is constricted. I may have difficulties talking or breathing. But I cannot connect these sensations to my emotions. I often wonder why it has to be so hard, why I feel invisible, and why it hurts so bad. I often feel taken for granted and unappreciated, stuck in one-sided family relationships, friendships, and romances. Alone.

I usually don't let myself feel anything long enough to be able to name it. Instead, I eat and disconnect myself from it. My physical responses to my feelings sometimes catch up with me: anxiety feels like a lump in my throat, anger feels like shouting at the top of my lungs, fear feels like a cold bowling ball in my stomach. So I do my best to also cut myself off from any physical sensation, and I stop paying attention to my body too. I neglect all aspects of myself in order to not feel anything. I become a simple witness of what happens to me.

If I don't feel anything, I don't hurt. I don't lie when I say, "I'm fine."

My extra weight is the sand in the gears. This visible "detail" uncovers my obvious lie when I say, "I am fine." My body expresses how unfulfilled I am since I don't allow myself to *feel* unfulfilled. My extra pounds show I am not fine in spite of the big smile on my face. I don't eat far beyond my energetic needs, and I don't put my life at risk, because I am "fine." I eat to not feel the pain I live with. I eat instead of working toward being "fine."

I know something is wrong with my way of life, but I don't know what, and I sure don't know what to do to make it right.

If I decide to stop eating my emotions, what should I do when the emotional warning lights start flashing on the dashboard of my inner self? Emotional eating has allowed me to function pretty well with those warning lights constantly flashing for such a long time. In spite of them, I am able to hold onto a job, pay my bills on time, and people seem to think I am fun and likable. I am afraid of what I might learn if I check why those lights are still on after all these years.

The more my emotional lights are flashing at me, the busier I get in order to ignore them. I binge-watch another TV show (preferably with at least a bag or two of cookies), scroll on my social media all night long, and keep my social calendar very full. I dive deep into work and convince myself being more productive and successful will fill that void in my life. I distract myself from those flashing lights in every possible way—food being my favorite.

My emotional warning lights do not always mean something is wrong. Many times, they are a way to teach me about a false belief I have embraced about myself. They show me where I am trying to find my significance and remind me where my true identity is found. They simply reveal me for who I am, not who I want to be. I learn about myself when I listen to my emotions, and I start asking myself real questions, like, why am I so anxious? What exactly am I crying over? What makes me so angry? Why do I stay in dysfunctional relationships? Why am I constantly worried? Why do I keep myself so distracted? Why do my thoughts keep on waking me up at night? Why can't I just believe in myself? What does that even mean?

My emotions are a gauge, not a guide. They are not a GPS.

They are designed to *read* my inner self, not to *lead* it. If I want to be real, I have to embrace the real me, which includes my thoughts, intentions, choices, and feelings. Not only the superficial ones, but also the deep ones: love, joy, emptiness, fear, sadness, sorrow, and my overwhelming anger. My emotions serve a purpose. Their purpose is to report information to me, to communicate what is going on behind my big smile.

Every emotion reveals a belief I have of what I am and of what I want. Every emotion can reveal where I have placed my identity, my significance, and my value. When I understand the information I am given, it is up to me to decide what I am going to do with it. As long as I eat my emotions and stay disconnected from them, I don't understand what I feel or why I feel it. I cannot adjust how I live and how I relate with others according to what I truly need and who I truly am. Every time I eat my emotions, I escape my feelings instead of giving myself what my emotions tell me I need. I deny myself the right to meet my needs.

Anger, fear, depression, and grief are said to be negative. But those feelings serve me when they tell me something is wrong in my life and needs to be corrected. Those feelings are healthy, positive responses in a situation that is hurtful to me and encourages me to devalue myself. I finally become more authentic when I listen to what I feel; my actions, thoughts, motivations, and words begin to align.

This is also when I don't need to eat my emotions as much as I used to. My anger, my shame, my pleasure, my pain, my joy, my anxiety, my boredom, and my despair help reveal my values, my motivations, my strengths, and my needs. If I don't know myself, I cannot know why I react as I do to my circumstances. I cannot distinguish the fear that says I am in danger from the fear that arises when faced with the need to change.

Today, I no longer see my depression, grief, anxiety, and anger as enemies.

Even when my emotions go off unwillingly, invading my body and my mind, they are not negative or positive by themselves. They just go through me, and they can be pleasant or unpleasant to experience. I try to treat them as messengers, sent to caution me, to remind me of my need for self-care, to help me reassess and release my attachments, to encourage me to reexamine my values, and to suggest it is time to revisit and revise the story of my identity.

As I listen to them, I can make the adjustments I need in my life. I can tell when I am where I am supposed to be because my difficult feelings are immediately replaced with balance and joy. My emotions are not a threat to me. Just the opposite; they are my rescuer.

The Challenge: Un-decoded and Unmet Emotional Needs

As humans, we seek emotional nourishment as much as food and water. Meeting our physical needs means we can stay alive, but it takes more to give life meaning. Emotional needs are feelings or conditions we need to feel happy, fulfilled, or at peace. Emotional needs have a lot to do with relationships, and some examples might include feelings of being appreciated, accomplished, safe, or part of a community. We can't see or touch things like companionship, affection, security, or appreciation, but they are just as valuable as feeling heard or valued. Without them, we may feel frustrated, hurt, or dissatisfied.

There are five broad categories of emotional needs.

1. **To feel safe, stable, nurtured, and accepted.** These are the most fundamental of our core emotional needs.

   - We need a safe place: an environment that enables us to lead our lives without experiencing undue fear and that allows us to develop our potential.

   - Stability is about having a basic level of predictability or routine in our life and knowing we have people around us available for support and connection.

   - Nurturance includes attention, affection, warmth, and companionship. It is about feeling protected, cared for, and guided by others.

   - To be accepted by others is to feel as though we are likable, lovable, and worthwhile as a person.

2. **To have some autonomy, to feel competent, and to have a sense of identity.** We need to feel as if we have the power to exist autonomously and direct our own lives.

3. **To have the freedom to express our own needs and emotions.** When we don't feel free to express our needs and emotions, we suppress our spontaneous feelings, impulses, and choices by eating as a way to meet rigid, internalized rules and expectations about our performance and ethical behavior. Performance, duty, perfectionism, following the rules, hiding our emotions,

and avoiding mistakes take precedence over pleasure, joy, and relaxation. We put an excessive emphasis on gaining approval, recognition, or attention from other people, or on fitting in, at the expense of developing a secure and true sense of self. Our sense of self-esteem is dependent primarily on the reactions of others rather than on our own natural inclinations. Instead of our needs, we may focus on status, appearance, social acceptance, money, or achievement as means of gaining approval, admiration, or attention.

4. **To be able to act spontaneously and to play.** Our free will sometimes manifests itself in unplanned ways. We usually inhibit our spontaneous action, feeling, or communication to avoid disapproval by others, feelings of shame, losing control of our impulses, or feeling vulnerable. The most common areas of inhibition involve

- inhibition of anger and aggression,

- inhibition of positive impulses (such as joy, affection, sexual excitement, play),

- difficulty expressing vulnerability or communicating freely about our feelings, needs, and other aspects, and

- excessive emphasis on rationality while disregarding our emotions.

5. **To live in a world with realistic limits, which helps us to apply self-control.** When we are not given adequate supervision, direction, or guidance as children, we may tolerate abnormal levels of discomfort as adults. Growing up with impaired limits may create issues setting personal boundaries with others, as well as expressing our emotions in a safe and healthy way.

Emotional needs are not set in stone. As we mature and learn more about ourselves, we might have different needs throughout our life, and our needs can also shift within one specific relationship. For example, we don't have the same needs from our parents when we are adults as we did when we were children. We may need something different in our relationship with our significant other after some time spent together too.

Everyone has their own unique set of emotional needs, which might be the product of our upbringing, our genetic predisposition, our identity, and other individual factors. Some people might value belonging over love, or trust over desire, for example. While some of us might prioritize certain traits, such as attention and connectedness, some others might place more importance on privacy and independence.

What Happens When Our Emotional Needs Are Not Met?

When our emotional needs are not met, it leads to emotional suffering. Water, sunlight, air, and nutrients are the core needs for healthy plant life. In the same way, we must have our core emotional needs met to be mentally and emotionally healthy. Just as wilted leaves are the first signs that a plant is not thriving, there are signs when our core emotional needs are not being met adequately. In her article "The five signs of emotional suffering", Jodi Gilman describes the main signs of emotional suffering. She mentions:

- exhibiting a personality change that could have occurred a long time ago, depending on when the distress started (for example, as a toddler, I suddenly turned from extroverted to introverted);

- being agitated or anxious;

- being withdrawn socially or in relationships with others;

- having poor self-care;

- feeling hopeless; and

- living in a cluttered environment.

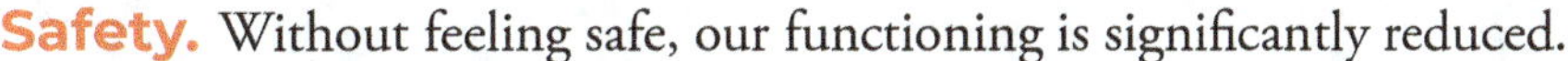

Not meeting our emotional needs leads to a significant decrease in our well-being in these areas:

Safety. Without feeling safe, our functioning is significantly reduced.

Stability. When we feel the people around us are emotionally unstable and unpredictable (example: angry outbursts), unreliable, or erratically present, or they may leave us in favor of someone better or a better situation, we may develop fear and a feeling of abandonment.

Nurturance. Without sufficient nurturing from others as children and as adults, we have to rely too heavily on ourselves, and this may lead us to develop bouts of sadness and depression.

Acceptance by others. When we feel like we are ignored, we may develop a sense of defectiveness and feel we are bad, inferior, invalid, unimportant, or unlovable.

Autonomy and competency. When we lack a feeling of autonomy, we may feel like we are not in control of our life. We may believe we are unable to handle our everyday responsibilities (such as taking care of ourselves, solving daily problems, exercising good judgment, tackling new tasks, making good decisions) in a competent manner without considerable help from others. We may develop a feeling of helplessness, have issues making responsible choices that include eating choices, and have difficulties setting clear boundaries in our relationships with others. In more severe deprivation of this needs fulfillment, we may believe we cannot survive or be happy without the constant support of someone else, or we may experience a feeling of emptiness and floundering.

Freedom to express our needs and emotions. When we feel like we cannot express our feelings and needs without suffering negative consequences, we may make life decisions that are inauthentic or unsatisfying. This may lead us to feel disconnected in our relationships with others and can have a negative impact on our feeling of happiness, our ability to relax, our eating behavior, and our health in general. We may feel pessimistic and worry things could fall apart if we fail to be vigilant and careful at all times. We may also experience a constant feeling of walking on eggshells.

Spontaneity and play. When we feel like we cannot pursue something we suddenly want or have fun in an unexpected moment because we believe it would not be appropriate, we may lose our sense of individuality and the meaning in our life.

Realistic limits. Impaired limits may lead us to feel an increased sense of responsibility toward others at the expense of the respect of our own rights, and we may have a tendency to set unrealistic personal goals. Impaired limits also cause us to create self-defeating patterns and to self-sabotage.

When our core emotional needs are not being met adequately, we are emotionally starving. In a maladaptive attempt to cope, we try to fill our stomach, which brings a temporary sense of relief, but doesn't help us feel better because our starvation is not physical but emotional.

 *Our Unmet Emotional Needs Directly Impact How We Feel*

Life is never 100 percent perfect, but as long as our essential needs are being met, no need to eat our emotions exists. However, if just one of our core needs is unmet, the void can lead us to emotional eating. From that perspective, recognizing our emotions is important. Recognition allows us to use how we feel to identify our unmet emotional needs. Our emotions are like our internal compass, helping us figure out how a situation makes us feel. When we know how a situation makes us feel, we know whether it contributes to fulfilling our emotional needs or not, and we can make the decision to stay in that situation or not.

Our feelings tell us some situations are not right for us. If we are able to listen to our feelings, we will be more likely to gravitate toward people who contribute to fulfilling our emotional needs. If we do not have this awareness, we may not even realize some people around us may have a negative impact on our well-being, and the simple decision to stay in certain situations feeds our emotional eating.

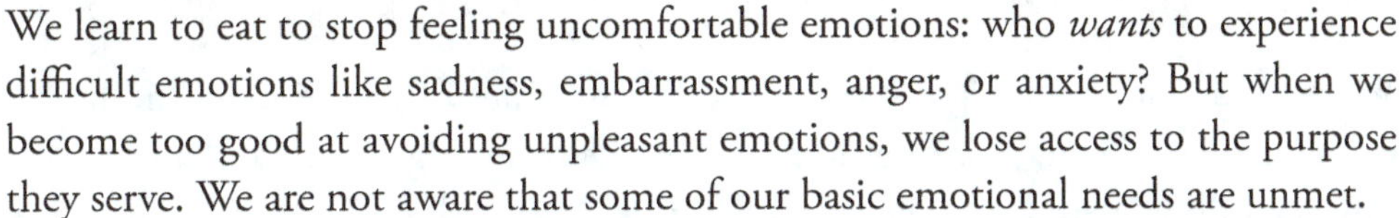

We naturally and automatically move toward what feels good and away from what feels bad.

We learn to eat to stop feeling uncomfortable emotions: who *wants* to experience difficult emotions like sadness, embarrassment, anger, or anxiety? But when we become too good at avoiding unpleasant emotions, we lose access to the purpose they serve. We are not aware that some of our basic emotional needs are unmet.

Reversing the process and learning to name our feelings does not come naturally, and we may sometimes find it difficult to name what we feel. But when we are able to decode our emotions, we can do the following:

- Make decisions more easily. When we understand what we feel and why we feel it, we are able to decide what to do to make the feeling last longer if we like it or to cut it short if we don't.

- Take action to change an emotionally taxing situation.

- Allow others to understand us and offer us the support we may need.

We eat on autopilot every time we feel something uncomfortable. It takes an assumed willingness to listen to our authentic emotions to override our emotional eating and stop coping with our unmet needs through eating. When we intentionally allow ourselves to feel and name our uncomfortable feelings instead of eating them, we can meet the emotional needs that activated them.

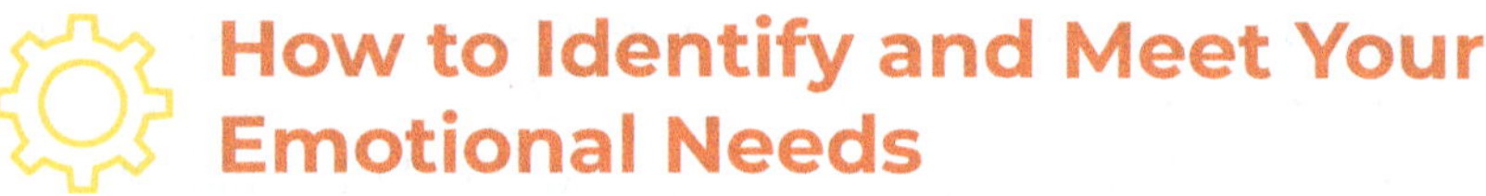

How to Identify and Meet Your Emotional Needs

All of us have emotional needs, but what fulfills each of us can vary. A need appears when we lack something, when we are denied something essential to our life. Instead of giving ourselves what we need, we have learned not to pay attention to how we feel when our needs are unmet. We have developed many strategies and beliefs to keep us away from our emotions "for our own good" so we don't change or walk away from the dissatisfying situations we find ourselves in. Emotional eating is our favorite one but not the only one.

Our will to "control" our emotions makes us forget we don't have that power. In the same way we cannot control the weather outside, we cannot control our emotions and the "weather inside."

Determine Your Main Emotional Needs

Your emotional needs might change at different times in your life depending on what happens to you. This questionnaire will help you highlight your current top three emotional needs. Keep in mind that this is a snapshot of today's needs. Your needs can change over time and circumstances, and you can retake this test as many times as you want as a way to check where you stand.

→ **Please rate the following affirmations by circling the number you think is most true for you at the moment:**

-2 = This is never true for me.

-1 = This is not really true for me.

0 = I do not know.

1 = This is sometimes true for me.

2 = This is always true for me.

1	It is important that people like me for who I am, even if I seem to be a little different.
	-2 -1 0 1 2

2	It is important to me that I can manage my finances.
	-2 -1 0 1 2

3	I sometimes become tired and worn down by looking after others.
	-2 -1 0 1 2

4	It is really important to me for people to ask my opinion even on small things.
	-2 -1 0 1 2

5	It is really important I receive hugs, cuddles, and strokes.
	-2 -1 0 1 2

6	I feel good when someone gives me time and listens, so I know they understand.
	-2 -1 0 1 2

7	I feel pleased when people tell me I have done well.
	-2 -1 0 1 2

8	I like it when people notice I need help and then offer it.
	-2 -1 0 1 2

9	When I have too much to cope with, I like someone to come alongside and help.
	-2 -1 0 1 2

10	I feel special when someone shows they know how I am feeling.
	-2 -1 0 1 2

11	I like to think people value me for the kind of person I am.
	-2 -1 0 1 2

12	It is important that I can express my thoughts and feelings.
	-2 -1 0 1 2

13	I love it when someone tells me, "I love you."
	-2 -1 0 1 2

14   I like to be seen as an individual—not just one of a group.

| -2 | -1 | 0 | 1 | 2 |

15   I like it when a friend calls and listens to me, then tells me I am doing a good job and to keep going.

| -2 | -1 | 0 | 1 | 2 |

16   I like people to praise me for who I am and not just for the things I do.

| -2 | -1 | 0 | 1 | 2 |

17   I like it when things are predictable and ordered.

| -2 | -1 | 0 | 1 | 2 |

18   When I work hard on someone's behalf, I like them to say thank you.

| -2 | -1 | 0 | 1 | 2 |

19   When I make a big mistake and "blow it," it's important to me that people forgive me and still love me.

| -2 | -1 | 0 | 1 | 2 |

20   I like it when other people notice what I have done.

| -2 | -1 | 0 | 1 | 2 |

21   I sometimes feel completely overwhelmed with all that needs to be done.

| -2 | -1 | 0 | 1 | 2 |

22   I want to be treated with kindness and respect whatever my race, gender, beliefs, looks, or what I have done or not done in my life.

| -2 | -1 | 0 | 1 | 2 |

23   All my friends and family know I like a good hug.

| -2 | -1 | 0 | 1 | 2 |

24   I like it when those close to me want to spend time with me.

| -2 | -1 | 0 | 1 | 2 |

25   I am pleased when my boss or another person in authority tells me I have done a good job.

| -2 | -1 | 0 | 1 | 2 |

26	It is important someone shows they care if I am having a bad day.
	-2 -1 0 1 2

27	When I am in a difficult time, I really like other people to do something practical to support me.
	-2 -1 0 1 2

28	If I were bereaved or very upset, I would like it if someone wrote me a note saying they sympathize with me.
	-2 -1 0 1 2

29	It is important I know whether people like me or not.
	-2 -1 0 1 2

30	I like it when people praise me in front of others.
	-2 -1 0 1 2

31	I really like it when someone reaches out to hold my hand or pat my shoulder.
	-2 -1 0 1 2

32	I don't like people who try to control me and tell me what to do.
	-2 -1 0 1 2

33	I feel pleased when someone is interested in what I am doing.
	-2 -1 0 1 2

34	I like a certificate or something that reminds me of something I have done or achieved.
	-2 -1 0 1 2

35	I want my partner, friends, and family to be there for me "through thick and thin."
	-2 -1 0 1 2

36	When I meet new people, it is important they like me.
	-2 -1 0 1 2

37	I don't like it when things change.
	-2 -1 0 1 2

38	I don't like prejudice of any kind.
	-2 -1 0 1 2

39 | I often worry about the future.
-2   -1   0   1   2

40 | I like it when people write me notes saying thank you and telling me what I did that they were pleased with.
-2   -1   0   1   2

41 | When someone tells me they have been thinking of me, it really means a lot to me.
-2   -1   0   1   2

42 | When decisions are made about me or my family, I like to be part of making them.
-2   -1   0   1   2

43 | I like to be greeted with a kiss, hug, or handshake depending on how well I know someone.
-2   -1   0   1   2

44 | I like it when people spend time with me alone and just concentrate on me.
-2   -1   0   1   2

45 | I like people close to me to tell me my special qualities.
-2   -1   0   1   2

46 | I respond to someone who tries to understand me and shows me concern and compassion.
-2   -1   0   1   2

47 | I prefer to work on things with someone else—two heads are better than one.
-2   -1   0   1   2

48 | It is important to me to feel part of any group I am in and not an outsider.
-2   -1   0   1   2

49 | I don't like to be alone when I am upset or in trouble. I need those I love around me or at least keeping in touch.
-2   -1   0   1   2

50 | I would rather work as part of a team than on my own.
-2   -1   0   1   2

→ Now, let's put your score sheet together. For each emotional need listed below, please add up the answers to the question numbers listed, then record your total in the space provided.

EMOTIONAL NEED	QUESTION NUMBER	TOTAL
Acceptance	1, 19, 36, 38, 48	
Affection	5, 13, 23, 31, 43	
Appreciation	18, 20, 25, 34, 40	
Approval	7, 11, 16, 29, 45	
Attention	6, 12, 24, 30, 44	
Comfort	10, 26, 28, 46, 49	
Encouragement	3, 15, 21, 33, 41	
Respect	4, 14, 22, 32, 42	
Security	2, 17, 35, 37, 39	
Support	8, 9, 27, 47, 50	

All of our emotional needs have to be met for us to be balanced. While we can manage to see the less important of them unmet for a short period of time, when our most essential ones are not met, it creates an immediate distress and activates emotional eating.

→ The needs that score the highest in the previous table are the more important ones for you right now. What are your three most important emotional needs as of today?

____

____

Congratulations! You just made a big leap into self-awareness. Knowing what you need the most will help you keep yourself fulfilled. The more fulfilled your needs are, the less you will have to compensate for unmet needs with food. Great job!

# *Assess Your Level of Emotional Fulfillment*

All of us have emotional needs that cannot be avoided. How inclined we are to eat our emotions depends on how well those needs are being met and how well we deal with the situation when they are not being met.

Please rate how well you perceive that the following emotional needs are being met in your life as of today, on a scale of 1 to 10, where 1 means not met at all and 10 means being totally met.

➔ **How secure do you feel today in the major areas of your life? (For example, your home, work environments.)**

1	2	3	4	5	6	7	8	9	10

➔ **What level of attention do you feel you receive most of the time?**

1	2	3	4	5	6	7	8	9	10

➔ **How in control of your life do you feel most of the time?**

1	2	3	4	5	6	7	8	9	10

➔ **To what extent do you feel part of a wider community?**

1	2	3	4	5	6	7	8	9	10

➔ **How often can you obtain privacy when you need to?**

1	2	3	4	5	6	7	8	9	10

➔ **To what extent do you feel an emotional connection to others?**

1	2	3	4	5	6	7	8	9	10

➔ **To what extent do you feel your status is acknowledged?**

1	2	3	4	5	6	7	8	9	10

→ To what extent do you feel like you are achieving things and that you are competent in at least one major area of your life?

1   2   3   4   5   6   7   8   9   10

→ To what extent do you feel mentally or physically stretched in ways that give you a sense of meaning and purpose?

1   2   3   4   5   6   7   8   9   10

If you currently are involved in a romantic relationship, please focus on it to answer the next set of questions. If you are currently not in a romantic relationship, please focus on one relationship that is currently meaningful to you (friendship, fraternal, or sisterly relationship) to answer:

→ How happy are you with this situation?

1   2   3   4   5   6   7   8   9   10

→ How much do you feel appreciated and valued in this relationship?

1   2   3   4   5   6   7   8   9   10

→ To what extent do you feel like your partner's, friend's, or sibling's top priority?

1   2   3   4   5   6   7   8   9   10

→ To what extent do you feel wanted and desired in this relationship?

1   2   3   4   5   6   7   8   9   10

→ To what extent do you feel honored and respected in this relationship?

1   2   3   4   5   6   7   8   9   10

→ To what extent do you feel seen and accepted in this relationship?

1   2   3   4   5   6   7   8   9   10

→ **To what extent does this relationship bring you a deep sense of emotional connection?**

1   2   3   4   5   6   7   8   9   10

→ **To what extent do you feel completely accepted for who you are in this relationship?**

1   2   3   4   5   6   7   8   9   10

If your scores are mostly low (5 or below), you are more likely to be inclined to emotional eating to manage the stress associated with your unmet emotional needs.

If any need is scored 3 or lower, this is likely a major stressor for you and therefore a major factor of emotional eating.

Even if only one need is marked very low, it can be enough of a problem to induce stress, anxiety, anger, or depression and seriously influence your emotional eating.

→ **What do your scores look like? Do they tend to be high, average, or low? Which ones are really high? Which ones are really low? How do your scores make you feel?**

Some of these situations are not always easy to evaluate. Whenever you're unsure how to answer, just give yourself a little time to fully process the question. If you feel an uncomfortable emotion or body sensation as you read a question, it may mean that a part of you may be reluctant to answer honestly because the answer doesn't please you. It is a totally normal reaction.

In that case, you may want to reflect on what causes your reaction before you answer the question, and why you feel the way you feel about it. Remember, self-judgment is counterproductive. Facing the reality of where you are today will help you make your peace with emotional eating, and from there, you will be able to bring positive change to your relationship with food.

 ## *Take Action to Meet Your Emotional Needs*

Our emotions signal a need. When something is important to us, we are supposed to feel emotions. Each emotion informs us of what we value and what we need. When we learn to truly listen to the emotion that is currently primary for us, we are listening to the needs of our authentic self. Our emotional response to an event is a way to ensure our safety, provide information about what we need, and get our needs met in our relationships with others.

During childhood, we rely on our parents (or the people who raised us) for our emotional needs—love, comfort, support, validation, as examples. As adults, some of us, including me, still tend to want someone else to make us happy, blame others for our unhappiness, and seek to fulfill our emotional needs through others. As we do so, we get exposed to

- relationship problems, because if the other person does not meet our needs, we resent it;

- being unhappy, because we think happiness is outside of us and depends on someone or something else, and therefore is unreliable and elusive; and

- feeling helpless, because if other people are supposed to make us happy and fulfill our needs, then what can we do if they don't?

We eat our emotions because we have become reliant on outside reinforcement to tell us how we should feel and what we should need and care about.

But our internal experience is the only thing that can connect us to what we need and remind us to do what is necessary to fulfill it. A need that is not met creates negative emotions, anxiety, and stress. When we eat our emotions, we eat so we don't take action and so we don't change what is unfulfilling in our lives because it would go against what is expected of us.

Together with the loss of connection to others and the loss of motivation to take action, eating our emotions mutes our awareness of what is important to us, what we lack, and what we need. We lose sight of what we truly need, and we become more prone to make decisions based on outside demands rather than on our own needs. When we prioritize what is expected from us over what we need, our emotional needs are unmet, and we find comfort in emotional eating.

We highlighted your emotional needs and how well met they are in the previous exercise. Now, let's think about how you can have them better met. Please consider your important emotional needs today as you identified them in the two sections above.

➜ **What makes you feel not enough** ______________________ (need #1) **today?**

____

➜ **What do you need to feel more** ______________________ (need #1) **today?**

____

➜ **What first step can you take today toward this goal?**

____

➜ **What makes you feel not enough** ______________________ (need #2) **today?**

____

➜ **What do you need to feel more** ______________________ (need #2) **today?**

____

➜ **What first step can you take today toward this goal?**

____

➜ **What makes you feel not enough** ______________________ (need #3) **today?**

____

➜ **What do you need to feel more** ______________________ (need #3) **today?**

____

➜ **What first step can you take today toward this goal?**

____

You can repeat this exercise with every one of your emotional needs, especially the ones you feel are currently unmet.

Emotions motivate action impulses. Each emotion has a unique footprint that conveys fast-acting yet subtle bodily sensations. We experience them as impulses to take a necessary action to get our needs met. When we stay connected to what we feel and are able to put words on our emotions, we can take action to meet our needs. When we do so, eating as a coping mechanism does not have a function anymore; if we take action when we need something, there is no unmet need left to cope with.

Jump-Start

→ **When was the last time that you were anxious? What happened?**

→ **How did you know you were anxious? What physical sensations did you experience? How did you behave?**

→ **What would you have needed not to feel anxious or to drastically reduce your level of anxiety?**

→ **When was the last time you were angry? What happened?**

→ **How did you know you were angry? What physical sensations did you experience? How did you behave?**

➡ **What would you have needed not to feel angry or to drastically reduce your level of anger?**

➡ **When was the last time you were upset or depressed? What happened?**

➡ **How did you know you were upset or depressed? What physical sensations did you experience? How did you behave?**

➡ **What would you have needed not to feel upset or depressed or to drastically reduce your level of sadness?**

➡ **What do you lack today in your life (time, attention, desire, surprise, something else)?**

➡ **What was the last actual good time you had? What happened?**

→ **How did you feel?**

→ **What specific component(s) of these happy moments made you feel good?**

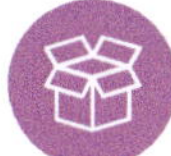 ## *Thinking Outside the Box*

Accurately labeling our emotions is a psychological superpower. It transforms a murky experience like "stress" into a finite one with boundaries and a name like "disappointed" or "depleted." It enables you to effectively move forward toward your needs and values.

This is a coaching exercise meant to help you focus on how you feel and to help you describe it using the metaphor of the weather. The more you practice this exercise, the more you become able to connect to and put into words how you feel.

Please, get comfortable and take a few deep breaths.

→ **What is the weather like inside of you?**

Example: Warm and bright sunny day, cloudy, rainy, stormy, tornado, changing weather, fog, icy, flooding, high wind, frost advisory.

Getting back in touch with our feelings is a process, especially if we have been disconnected from them for a long time. If you cannot tell how you feel, make a full body and sensory scan.

→ On a scale from 1 to 10, 1 for the minimum and 10 for the maximum, how is your energy level?

1   2   3   4   5   6   7   8   9   10

→ What can you feel?

Example: I am tired, hungry, squeamish, weak, energized, something else.

____

____

→ What does your body tell you?

Example: I feel light/heavy, I feel tense, my back is hurting.

____

____

→ What ideas are crossing your mind?

Example: Projects, positive or negative thoughts, something else.

____

____

→ What feelings/emotions are you experiencing right now? (There can be several at the same time.)

Example: I feel irritated and somewhat nervous.

____

____

→ What is the most prominent of these feelings?

Try to investigate past answers like "fine" or "okay," and ask yourself what "fine" means, for example.

Example: I feel nervous. I feel content.

____

____

→ When did you become aware of this feeling?

Example: Right now.

____

____

→ Using your body as a scale like you were a living emotional barometer going from 1 to 10, identify up to what level your emotion is filling you up, from the bottom up.

Example: I am at 7, up to my shoulders. I am at 2, up to my knees.

____

____

→ What might be triggering this feeling?

Example: I am nervous because I facilitated an important meeting at work today, and I still have not heard from my boss about it.

____

____

If no obvious answer comes up after completing this body scan, you might try asking yourself what is happening (or not happening) in your current life.

→ How do you get along with your partner, children, parents, and siblings?

Try to investigate past answers like "fine" or "okay," and ask yourself what "fine" means, for example.

____

____

➔ **How are you doing at work? How much do you enjoy work and get along with your coworkers and your boss?**

Try to investigate past answers like "fine" or "okay," and ask yourself what "fine" means, for example.

____

____

➔ **Notice if you start judging what you feel.**

Example: I don't have any reason to feel anxious; my boss is probably busy.

____

____

➔ **Push those judgments away and take a few deep breaths. What do you need?**

Example: I need to move, I need a hug, I need to be paid more attention to.

____

____

➔ **Take a few more deep breaths. Notice how you feel now. Do you experience some change in your inner weather after this exercise? Has your emotional state stayed the same? Gotten stronger or weaker?**

____

____

This exercise allows you to put words to your feelings and the needs behind them. The more you train your brain not to judge your feelings, the more you feed self-empathy and allow yourself to make your relationship with yourself smoother. In addition, observing the emotions and sensations that come and go through you and accepting them as a part of yourself without judging them allows them to evolve, be tamed, or transform into something different. The more you can label your emotions without judging what you are feeling, the less you find them unacceptable and eat to mute them. You can practice this exercise as often as you want to.

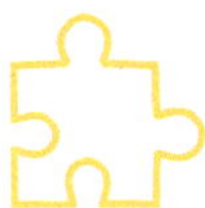

Takeaway

> *Emotions are celebrated and repressed, analyzed and medicated, adored and ignored—but rarely, if ever, are they honored."*

—*Karla McLaren*

You are already successful!

Congratulations! You made it through this important step. It was tough, but you pushed through it. Every time you engage in negative self-talk, please remember you've come this far, and there is no way you could have done this without willpower or a strong desire to bring positive and long-lasting change to your life.

In addition, you are probably not a total stranger to what we discussed in this chapter. That means you have been on your way to recovery for some time. Let's capitalize on your existing achievements and experience.

➜ **What have you already tried/started/accomplished in the area discussed in this chapter that previously worked/was a success/was promising?**

____

____

➜ **What happened to get you started?**

____

____

➜ **What was your recipe for success?**

____

____

➜ **How can you use this proven successful recipe today?**

____

____

 *Along the Path*

➔ **What have you been through while reading this chapter** *(what happened, how did you feel, what were your reactions, what important conversation did you have, did you have unusual dreams or body reactions/sensations)?*

➔ **What new perspective did you grasp in your relationship with food and with yourself or others or both?**

➔ **What new concept did you discover?**

➔ **What did you learn?**

➔ **What realization did you come to?**

➔ **What do you want to remember?**

Moving Forward

WHAT WILL YOU DO LESS?

✖

✖

✖

WHAT WILL YOU STOP DOING?

✖

✖

✖

WHAT WILL YOU START DOING?

✓

✓

✓

WHAT WILL YOU DO MORE OF?

✓

✓

✓

→ **Which one of these decisions will be the easiest for you to apply right now?**

You may feel what you have discovered and processed during this chapter is enough for you to successfully impact your relationship with food. This is great, and you are ready to jump into the next change. You may also feel it would be useful for you to dig deeper and explore these topics or some related areas a little bit more. If you want to take your reflection process and experimentation one step further, do this exercise.

WHAT ASPECTS DO YOU WANT TO EXPLORE MORE?   **HOW WILL YOU MAKE THIS EXPLORATION POSSIBLE?**

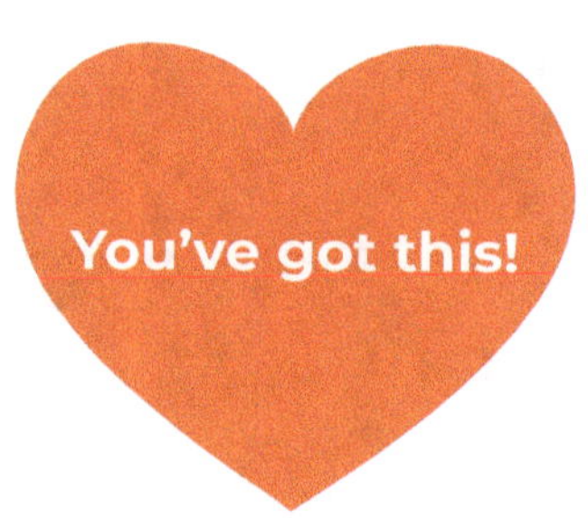

NOTES:

Express Your Feelings to Set Yourself Free

*Your Emotions Are Never
Too Intense to Be Released*

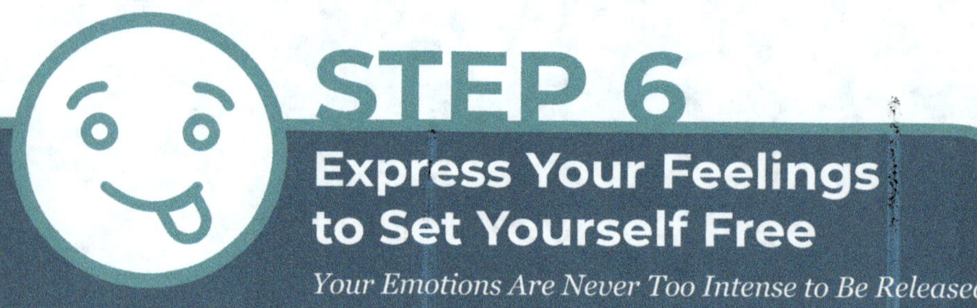

I don't understand what triggers my emotional eating. I don't see myself as emotionally repressed. My major issues belong to my past. As a child, my parents were under a great amount of stress and had plenty of adult issues to deal with. I became used to not being given the opportunity to express my feelings and my needs. I learned to stay passive and to censor myself so I could avoid trouble. My childhood was not great, but I sometimes wonder if what happened was really that bad or if I am just being dramatic.

Today, my life is about average. I get stressed about work issues; I sometimes get frustrated at home or with my friends, but who doesn't? My parents have not always been perfect, but I can deal with where I currently am in my relationships with them. The way I lead my career and my love life could be better, but I have a stable and decent life. I do not face any large struggles today. I feel as if I am not particularly different from anybody else. I am a happy-go-lucky person. I really am. I am always in a good mood, always smiling, and I have tons of friends! It's just when I am alone that I feel bored and uncomfortable. If I have to be by myself, I call or text people, or I binge watch television while snacking.

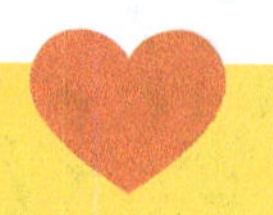

My life seems superficially balanced, but living a balanced life does not mean I am in balance myself.

Everything seems balanced in my life because I use food as a mood regulator. When I am faced with an uncomfortable situation, I don't talk about it. I don't try to fix it. I eat it. I just devour whatever trouble occurs. I maintain a precarious, sometimes delusional balance as I cultivate the appearance of calm and happiness. I try to look normal, and I contain my feelings behind my smile.

People around me are so used to me never asking for help and always putting their needs before mine they don't think about taking care of me either. They believe I am incredibly strong and always fine when I simply keep my emotions locked up, thanks to my best friend who is always there: food. Keeping my environment in balance is more important to me than keeping myself in balance or taking care of my own needs. I am about a hundred pounds overweight, but I tell myself my life is normal.

I don't let anyone know when they hurt me. I tell myself they don't deserve it, and I would give them too much power over me. But by staying quiet, I never get rid of the pain, the anger, the deception, and the grudges. I keep chaos inside. Not expressing anything has become so important that when I need to unleash my emotions and their violence, I sometimes turn them against myself.

When I feel disrespected and the need to get even, I don't want to let anger take control of my actions. I keep it all inside, and I get a sense of relief by hurting myself, basically eating until I hurt. My extra pounds physically materialize all the feelings that I have held onto. I truly want to lose weight, but sometimes I really need to eat to escape those raging inner monsters I am locked up with.

I mute my anger because I am afraid I could hurt someone if I express its real intensity. When I face the extent of my anger, I feel guilty. To be aggressive is not morally acceptable in my ethical beliefs. Therefore, I am a bad person, and it is wrong to feel that way. I cannot let violence out, so I stay stuck with it. Thankfully, the more I eat, the less I hear it.

I am also afraid that if I allow myself to experience sadness, I will fall into such a deep depression, I will never be able to get out of it.

My emotions are so powerful, I don't trust myself to express them to myself and others in an unharmful way. I feel like they would submerge me, and I would drown in them.

When my emotions are about to take over, I isolate myself to eat. It brings me some relief, and I don't feel as close to exploding. I believe that eating allows me to keep my emotions under control, but the truth is that even though repressed, my emotions rule my life. My fear keeps me from taking further steps toward others and from getting close to anyone; past rejection leads me to a life of emotional isolation as my guard is always up; anger makes me cynical and bitter; unresolved hurts convince me I am destined to be a lifelong victim having a second-rate and second-class kind of existence.

How do I get safe enough to be real? How do I get real enough to start to heal? How do I embrace the beautiful, the ugly, the embarrassing, the forgettable, the painful, and the shameful in myself and in my life? I have been judged and rejected so many times that this level of vulnerability terrifies me.

What I feel is what I feel. I don't have control over it. How I channel my emotions is my choice, though. I can choose to let fear, anger, guilt, and shame destroy me. I can drown deeper into silence until I completely disappear and forget about who I am forever. I can eat until I am permanently numbed and live my life like a robot: eat—go to work—eat—come home—eat—repeat.

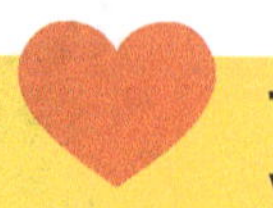

Today, I choose to fully express my emotions. I accept and confirm whatever I feel, whether I agree with it or not.

It is uncomfortable at first. Silenced for so long, my feelings come out strong and messy, but this does not last very long, and now I can state them peacefully. I have stopped holding onto my anger. Yes, my anger can be strong, but I never hurt anyone, physically or verbally. I learned how to express myself in an assertive way. My strong anger does not make me a bad person. My anger is simply this strong because I feel mistreated or disrespected. As I choose not to repress my feelings anymore, they don't control me, and I don't need to gobble them up anymore to mute them.

Being able to express my emotions allows me to choose the meaning I give to what I feel. The more I deal with them, the more I accept them as a part of who I am. To my surprise, nobody gets hurt in the process. Often, I actually find love and support to help me through them. When I let my feelings run their course through me, I am usually back to my normal self in a short period of time without the help of my precious food.

The situation that created my emotional state is not over, but I can ask myself why I feel this way. What is it that I need to feel better, and what action do I need to take to walk out of circumstances that are not good for me? As I dare express how I feel, I can finally be heard, at least by myself.

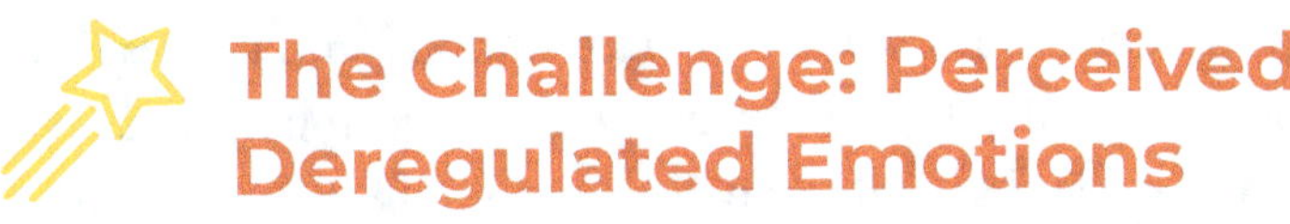

The Challenge: Perceived Deregulated Emotions

Psychology.com editors define emotional regulation as "the ability to influence our own emotions." It is the ability to respond to a situation using the full range of our emotions in a manner that is socially tolerable and sufficiently flexible to permit spontaneous reactions, as well as the ability to delay spontaneous reactions as needed. When we regulate our emotions, we are able to know what we feel and what to do about it in any environment. We are able to keep our emotions in balance and away from extremes.

When we are used to the people around us not favorably receiving the emotions we express, we believe the problem lies within us. We believe we are unable to control the manifestations of our emotions or moderate them according to what is socially acceptable.

When we think our emotions are deregulated, we believe we poorly modulate the way we react to social situations. When we express our feelings, we fear people around us find our emotional reactions inadequate, out of range, or unsuitable. So we start inhibiting our feelings.

The more we inhibit our emotions, the more it becomes difficult for us to

- be aware of, understand, and accept our emotional responses;
- take action to change a situation that upsets us;
- refrain from impulsive eating behaviors when we are upset; and
- express our feelings using the full range of emotional responses.

 *What We Do When We Believe Our Emotions Are Deregulated*

When we believe it is not appropriate to express our feelings, we simply suppress our emotions. This does not mean our feelings magically stop existing. The experience part of the emotion still persists; we still experience the emotion, but we inhibit its behavioral expression. This creates an asymmetry between how we feel and what others see. When they cannot see how we feel, they cannot take our emotions into account in the way they interact with us, and things may snowball.

Suppression only affects our behavioral response to our emotions, and it does little to reduce our actual experience. Therefore, suppressing our emotions comes at a high cost for us both cognitively and socially. It takes continuous effort to control and suppress our emotions, and that can create feelings of inauthenticity because we don't let others know our true feelings.

The more we suppress our emotions, the less we become able to repair our negative mood. We simply master the art of masking our inner feelings. Therefore, in the long run, suppressing our emotions leads us to experience

- fewer positive emotions,

- more negative emotions,

- less life satisfaction, and

- lower self-esteem.

Emotional eating is the instrument we use to inhibit our emotional response to what happens to us.

Signs That Suppressing Our Feelings Is Our Usual Way to Deal With Them

We actively suppress our feelings when we use four types of behaviors.

- We keep our emotions to ourselves.

- When we feel positive emotions, we are careful not to express them.

- We control our emotions by not expressing them.

- When we feel negative emotions, we make sure not to express them.

The following can be signs we actively "bottle up" our emotions.

- We feel uncomfortable around highly emotional people.

- We secretly think anger and sadness are bad.

- We rarely, if ever, cry or yell.

- If we do get angry or sad, we might overreact to something, a detail that may not be directly connected to what upsets us (for example, blowing up when we are asked to dry the dishes a little more carefully, when we are actually upset after a conversation with our partner).

- We think we feel fine all the time and see ourselves as laid back and easygoing.

- We heavily rely on escape behaviors like binge watching TV, playing video games for long periods of time, and oversleeping.

- We have experiences we are not sure we enjoy, but we just let them happen.

- Our thoughts essentially consist of negative thinking or criticism of ourselves and others (or both).

- We feel the need to be in control of things.

- Emotional eating accounts for the majority of our food intake.

Emotional suppression also shows up in the ways we relate to others, including these actions.

- We rarely (if ever) open up to people and prefer to be private.

- We might seem really open and easily chat with strangers, but the real "us" remains hidden.

- We might be the clown or the hit of a party, always making everyone else laugh, but we are still hiding our own feelings.

- We have few truly close friendships, and we struggle with intimacy; some of us may fear intimacy.

- If someone does something that bothers us, we say nothing and then plan to slowly back out of the relationship or secretly get back at them in our own time.

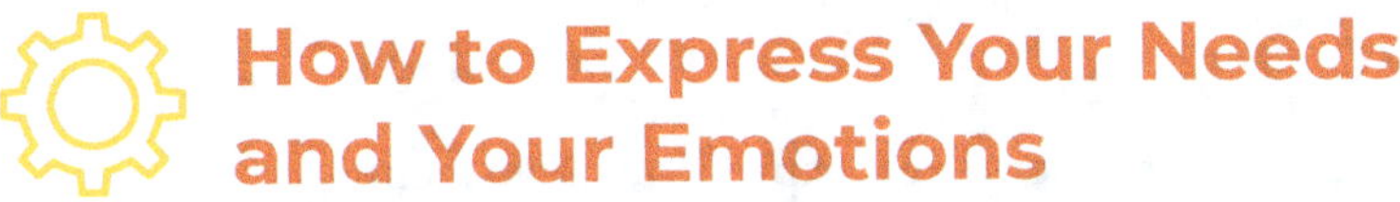

How to Express Your Needs and Your Emotions

We learned to focus on others and forget about what we feel inside. We learned getting angry is bad, so we need to be good and reasonable people. Expressing our emotions often is associated with weakness, and may simply feel wrong to us, so we do our best to look strong and look like we control our emotions. The truth is, we did not learn to control our emotions. That would require us to listen to them first. We simply learned to silence them.

The emotions we eat to bottle them up don't leave us as long as we don't express them. They only call out for us louder and louder. Emotions are meant to be expressed. They will not leave us alone as long as we refuse to oblige. We cannot stop eating our emotions as long as we don't allow them to be expressed. Their only mission is to be heard so that we can act accordingly and finally meet our emotional needs. Sometimes, eating them is no longer enough to silence them, and anxiety, sadness, or anger submerge us anyway.

If we decide to stop using food as a mood regulator and a quick fix to contain our emotions, we need to know how to handle and express them.

Identify Your Emotional Triggers

Since the first time we numbed ourselves with food to suppress our emotions, we've used emotional eating as our tool for dealing with them. Every time we eat our emotions, we add to the unprocessed feelings we carry. This means that when one emotion is even slightly activated in our everyday life, we react to it with the intensity born of all accumulated suppression of this same emotion.

Even if today's incident looks like a negligible event and seems easily manageable, we cannot handle it because we react too intensely. For example, expressing my anger is difficult for me. I repressed it so many times that I carry a huge amount of unprocessed anger. Today, I can get enraged over little things that should simply be minor irritants. I am afraid if I unleash my anger, it will get out of my control and I may become destructive or violent. So every time I start feeling the very beginning of irritation, I rush to food and numb it because losing control really scares me.

Suppressing our emotions gives us a way to control our current situation. When we are uncomfortable, embarrassed, and sometimes even scared to express our emotions, we may

- be scared to disappoint others if we express negative feelings,

- think we are going to bother others by showing them parts of ourselves we consider weaknesses,

- be scared to be submerged with the emotion or unleash it too intensely, or

- not want to fall apart and be forced to admit how down and very bad we actually feel.

Here are my main emotional eating triggers: the feelings I refuse to listen to that stimulate my urge to eat *right now.* When I feel like this, I cannot stand it, and I eat to suppress the emotions associated with my internal state. Those emotions most often are anger, fear, sadness, and anxiety; sometimes the four of them combine at different levels of intensity.

Please check off the triggers you share with me and add those that apply to you and are not cited.

☐ I feel excluded, left out.

☐ I feel powerless.

☐ I feel unheard.

☐ I feel scolded.

☐ I feel judged.

☐ I feel blamed.

☐ I feel disrespected.

☐ I feel a lack of affection.

☐ I feel I cannot speak up.

☐ I feel lonely.

☐ I feel I cannot be honest.

☐ I feel ignored.

☐ I feel invisible.

☐ I feel targeted.

☐ I feel _______________.

☐ I feel _______________.

☐ I feel like "the bad guy."

☐ I feel forgotten.

☐ I feel unsafe.

☐ I feel unloved.

☐ I feel like it was unfair.

☐ I feel frustrated.

☐ I feel disconnected from others.

☐ I feel trapped.

☐ I feel a lack of passion.

☐ I feel uncared for, neglected.

☐ I feel manipulated.

☐ I feel controlled.

☐ I feel taken advantage of.

☐ I feel inferior.

☐ I feel _______________.

☐ I feel _______________.

➜ Recall a situation that triggered your emotional eating. What happened?

Example: I lost three pounds, and I am excited. I want to share my joy with my partner, who quashes my joy by reminding me how much weight I still have to lose to reach my goal weight.

➜ What made you suppress your feelings and decide to eat?

Example: I did not want them to know they hurt me.

➜ What trigger were you really reacting to?

Example: I felt unloved.

It is never inappropriate to express your emotions. You are entitled to express what you need. At some point, many of us stopped believing that was true. Why? What truly gets in our way? The image of ourselves we want to project? Our ideals? All the active social norms between us and the person we talk to? The high intensity of our feelings? Whatever it is, it is not as important as our well-being.

With this exercise, you listened to yourself first before listening to anything else. Depending on how long you have been muting your feelings, you might need some practice to get comfortable. Take all the time you need. You are worth it.

Decrease Your Dependency On Someone Else's Emotional State

When we live in an environment that does not allow us to have a strong sense of differentiated self, we externalize our sense of validation and self-worth. We depend on the people around us to tell us if we are good or bad, and we do not rely on our internal experience to tell us how we feel and what we need. It becomes difficult to trust that we even have our own needs or the right to ask for them to be met. In this context,

- we may deal with anxiety issues when we try to separate our own choices from other people's reactions. It becomes less emotionally challenging to simply follow what others want and to forget about what we feel and what we need, and

- emotional expression may seem risky, if not selfish. We learned that our role is to take care of the people around us. It is hard to find a balance between "you do you" and "I'll do me." Expressing an emotion or a need would make people we are supposed to take care of uncomfortable and might make us feel like we have failed them or somehow abandoned them.

We suppress our emotions because we learned our success, safety, or happiness is intrinsically tied to making other people successful or safe or happy. Whether they are our parents, family, partners, spouses, friends, or employers, we feel we cannot express emotions unless in reaction to their needs. We therefore downgrade our needs and mute our own emotions to meet their needs.

Here are some of the behaviors I display when I do not validate the way I feel and when I depend on other people's input to decide how I must feel and how I must behave. Please check the ones that apply to you, too, and add the ones that you use that are not listed.

☐ *I wait for someone else to say or do something so that I know how to react rather than creating initial responses that address my needs.*
Example: When I date someone, I wait for my family and friends to meet them and give their opinion before I decide to go further into a relationship with them, disregarding my own feelings toward them.

☐ *I wait or allow other people to define what is right for me to feel, say, or ask for.*

Example: When I get a 1 percent salary raise at work, I wait for my partner/spouse's reaction to decide whether I am happy about it or if I think it is not enough. If they are not happy, I embrace their frustration.

☐ *I feel anxious when I do not get external validation that I did something well.*

Example: I get really anxious when I send a report to my boss and don't get any feedback from them. I cannot decide by myself if my work is good or not, and I rely on their feedback: if they are happy with me, then I did well. As long as I don't know if they are happy with me, I stand on slippery ground.

☐ *I have an increased sense of responsibility and self-blame about things that go wrong in other people's thoughts, feelings, and behaviors.*

Example: When my mother expects me to call her at a precise time, and I cannot make it because I had an emergency at work, she quickly imagines the worst has happened to me and starts calling police stations and hospitals. When I call her a few hours later, she gets really upset with me. I think she feels so bad because of me, that it is all my fault, and I accept her blame.

☐ *I feel like I have to accept whatever comes my way from my partner/ parents/boss/friends, and I have no right to ask for anything different.*

Example: I am trying to lose weight, but my partner does not support me. Worse, they make fun of me and belittle me, saying I have no willpower and that my attempt to lose weight will fail anyway. I am hurt, but I think I should be happy and grateful to have them in my life, so I stay quiet.

____

____

____

Please think of one relationship (at work, a friend, family, or romantic relationship) that is important to you.

On a sliding scale from 1 to 10, 1 being not satisfied at all, and 10 being totally satisfied, how satisfied are you in that relationship regarding the following propositions?

➜ **I am able to trust and open up about who I really am.**

1   2   3   4   5   6   7   8   9   10

➜ **I feel that the other person really values what I go through.**

1   2   3   4   5   6   7   8   9   10

→ I feel the other person can provide me some support.

1   2   3   4   5   6   7   8   9   10

→ I feel the other person lets me define by myself what I go through.

1   2   3   4   5   6   7   8   9   10

→ I feel I can express some interest or affection for the other person.

1   2   3   4   5   6   7   8   9   10

→ What do you notice when you visualize your answers?

____

→ What would you like to see that relationship evolve into, for it to become more satisfying?

____

→ On a sliding scale from 1 to 10, 1 for not able at all, and 10 for totally able, how well do you feel able to assert yourself in this relationship today?

1   2   3   4   5   6   7   8   9   10

→ Ideally, what level of assertiveness would you like to be able to reach in this relationship?

1   2   3   4   5   6   7   8   9   10

→ How many points is the gap between those two last scores? _______________

→ What can you do right now to assert yourself just a little bit more in this relationship to reduce the gap by one point?

____

With these activities, you are training your capacity to rely on what you feel to make decisions and to take action, when you may have relied on external factors previously. Only you know what you need, and your body will send you the appropriate signals to guide you. All you have to do is to listen more to yourself and less to other people or external circumstances. It may trigger some negative reactions from people who are used to having their way with you, and their response may make you feel really uncomfortable. But remember: those who really love you will stick around. You can do it!

Neutralize Your Automatic Emotional Suppression Response

Sometimes we believe our emotions interfere with our thoughts, our relationships, and our everyday choices. In reality, it is the opposite: our thoughts, the choices we want to stick to in spite of how much we dislike them, and negative self-judgments interfere with our feelings and our ability to express our needs. The more reluctant we are to express our feelings, the more important it is to push forward and speak up so we can embrace the big picture of our lives, make new choices, and take new actions to feel better.

Dealing with uncomfortable feelings is a part of the human condition. In our daily lives, we all encounter conflict, stress, frustration, and pain. Emotional regulation helps us keep the expression of our emotions within what is socially acceptable, while still manifesting open reactions to what happens to us. By properly managing our emotions, we are able to respond to difficult situations in a way that is open and healthy for us and socially appropriate for our environment. But the regulation of an emotion is not the regulation of its manifestation. Controlling how we feel and the intensity of our feelings is not the same as controlling our reactions because of what we feel.

The outside world has been sending us some binding messages since we were born, telling us what we should feel, what we should need, and how we should behave. Because we badly needed the people around us to recognize and to love us, we gave these messages too much importance. We stopped listening to our needs and suppressed our emotions. No matter how we were feeling, and depending on what was expected from us, we created some automatic answers to certain situations. These automatic answers still influence our behaviors and choices today.

There are five main autopilots, also called drivers, which lead us to not listen to our needs, to mute our emotions, and to replace the action urge associated with it with the urge to eat. Identifying them lowers their power over us and allows us to become aware of the emotions we suppress so we can follow our natural urge for action without replacing it with emotional eating.

Here is a self-evaluation made of fifty affirmations to help you identify the drivers that have impacted your behaviors.

Please rate every affirmation from 0 to 4.

0 = This is not me.

1 = This may be me.

2 = This sometimes is me.

3 = This often is me.

4 = This is totally me.

	AFFIRMATIONS	RATING
1	I always feel that I am working against the clock.	
2	Making an effort is more important than the result I get.	
3	I think I have to take care of myself in life.	
4	Before I begin a task, I need all the information.	
5	It is important that others have a good opinion of me.	
6	Stress boosts me.	
7	I am always afraid to not measure up.	
8	I am very demanding of myself and of others.	
9	To be satisfied, I have to reach excellence.	
10	I am more accommodating than average in order to be appreciated.	
11	I cannot delegate because others are too slow and cannot perform the task as well as I can.	
12	I have to spend a lot of energy to get things done.	
13	I don't express my emotions.	

14	I must be perfect to be efficient.	
15	For my boss, I am always available, even when I am at home.	
16	I talk fast.	
17	I feel oppressed, and I am afraid I could blow up if I let myself go.	
18	I like to accomplish noble tasks.	
19	Facts, numbers, logic —these are the true values.	
20	People need to be told what they want to hear.	
21	I am tempted to interrupt people to finish their sentences for them.	
22	I have felt responsible for what happens to others for a long time.	
23	Intellectual exchange is the field where I feel comfortable.	
24	Accuracy at any cost is the price of my image.	
25	I like knowing a coworker needs me.	
26	I often say "Hurry," "Yes, yes," and "So what?"	
27	Others say I often complain.	
28	I like to approach situations and problems with logic.	
29	I must look like I know everything.	
30	I must be able to bend over backward.	
31	I often pace when I wait for something.	
32	People are attracted to me because they find me nice.	
33	I find it hard to trust people and completely open up.	
34	For me, a criticism is the sign of my incompetence.	
35	I like helping others.	
36	I often tap with my fingertips or my feet.	
37	I create confused situations where I feel stupid and powerless.	
38	The way others judge me for what I do matters to me a lot.	
39	I am convinced I am the best.	
40	I don't know how to say no.	
41	I move too fast; that's why I make inadvertent errors.	
42	Too much effort to answer all these questions!	
43	I feel safe if I don't get involved emotionally.	
44	As long as a task is not performed the way I pictured it, I will start it all over again.	
45	I like to act as a confidant.	

46	I cannot stay inactive, and I multitask if needed.	
47	My mother used to tell me, "With a little bit more effort you could________."	
48	During teamwork, I don't like when timing or the defined goals are not respected and when people digress.	
49	I expect my employees, coworkers, or friends to do exactly what I tell them.	
50	Answering these questions, I wonder if my answers match what is expected of me.	

➔ Now, let's put your score sheet together. For each driver listed below, please add up the answers to the question numbers listed, then record your total in the space provided.

DRIVER	QUESTION NUMBER	TOTAL
Be Strong	3, 8, 13, 18, 23, 28, 33, 38, 43, 48	/40
Hurry Up	1, 6, 11, 16, 21, 26, 31, 36, 41, 46	/40
Try Hard	2, 7, 12, 17, 22, 27, 32, 37, 42, 47	/40
Be Perfect	4, 9, 14, 19, 24, 29, 34, 39, 44, 49	/40
Please Others	5, 10, 15, 20, 25, 30, 35, 40, 45, 50	/40

The higher the score, the stronger the influence of that driver on our behavior and the more we tend to eat to suppress the emotions that we perceive make us appear in opposition to the driver.

➔ What are your two or three strongest drivers?

____

____

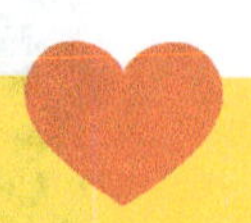 **Here are the mottos and feelings associated with each driver.**

Be Strong → Motto: *"I should not let others think I am weak."*

- When I score high for this driver, I tend to feel unappreciated and unable to get close to anybody.

- It leads me to carry heavy loads and put up with unbearable conditions. I tend to shut off my feelings and plow on, regardless of what is going on in my life; it is difficult to ask for what I want. Whatever I need, I get it myself.

- I need challenge.

- What I heard as a child: "You have to be brave," "What does not kill you makes you stronger," and "Big girls/boys don't cry."

Hurry Up → Motto: *"I am going to be late."*

- When I score high for this driver, I tend to feel like I don't belong, and I can panic quickly.

- I need to do everything fast. I rush things, even when it is not necessary and even when it would be better to take my time. I feel I am not good enough when I am not in a hurry.

- I need more time.

- What I heard as a child: "You are too slow" and "Stop dragging it out."

Try Hard → Motto: *"I am not working hard enough."*

- When I score high for this driver, I tend to feel like I don't get anywhere, and I constantly fear failure.

- It is the effort that matters. I feel okay when I work very hard, whether I accomplish something or not; at least I tried. I have a tendency to make things complicated and lose myself in details. I ponder the smallest things for a long time and often struggle to complete tasks and projects.

- I need to be paid more attention to.

- What I heard as a child: "Work harder" and "Victory without risk brings triumph without glory."

Be Perfect → Motto: *"I ought to be better."*

- When I score high for this driver, I tend to feel guilty, worthless, and anxious.

- I seek perfection in every way, and I maintain a completely flawless exterior. I put an enormous amount of effort into the details and will not settle until things are exactly right. I am not good enough if I happen to make a mistake. I will constantly try to improve myself in the hope of one day being accepted.

- I need to be recognized.

- What I heard as a child: "You can do better" and "It is not that bad, but I expected better from you."

Please Others → Motto: *"I earn love by taking care of others."*

- Taking care of others will make them appreciate me. I tend to see myself as responsible for what other people feel. I care more about their needs than my own. I like to keep everyone happy, often at my own expense.

- I need to feel loved.

- What I heard as a child: "Be nice with your mother/father/sibling," "You are hurting my feelings," "Don't be so selfish," and "Be kind, I am tired."

Most of the time, one or two drivers are clearly ahead of the others, but depending on how strong our environment has ruled our choices, it can be more.

→ How do your drivers contribute to your emotional eating?

Example: As I score high for the Be Strong driver, I tend to suppress my feeling of pain that I believe makes me weak. When a situation hurts me, I don't express it and don't let the other person know that they did me wrong. I stay impassible and eat to numb my pain and maintain the appearance that everything is fine with me.

To override our drivers and how they make us feel, we need to give ourselves permission to behave in a different way.

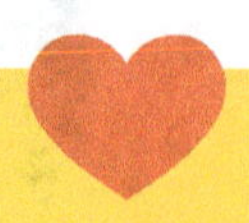

How to neutralize each driver.

Be strong

- I allow myself to ask for what I want and take care of my own needs.

- I have the right to have emotions. I can be myself. I can trust others. I can open up. I can enjoy daydreaming. I can talk to somebody.

Hurry Up

- I allow myself to slow down and take my time.

- I have the right to take my time. I can stay calm and still be efficient. I can let go sometimes. I can go far and at my own pace. I can manage my time.

Try Hard

- I allow myself to feel successful even if I do not work as hard as I can.

- I have the right to take my foot off the pedal. I can lower my ambitions. I can enjoy what I do. I can build smaller projects. I can define my own measure of success. I can replace effort with enjoyment.

Be Perfect

- I allow myself to feel good enough as I am; it is okay to be myself.

- I have the right to make mistakes; I can be human and simply be pleased with the work I accomplish. I can rejoice at the end of a task.

Please Others

- I allow myself to feel okay even if others are not happy with what I do.

- I have the right to express my wants, needs, and values. I can refuse what does not suit me. I can be more selfish. I can choose to work on my own personal projects. I can choose to be around people who make me feel good. I can let go of feeling responsible for others' feelings.

→ **What permission(s) do you give yourself today?**

Please be kind and patient with yourself; cancelling your autopilot modes can take some time to feel natural. Overriding your drivers takes practice. I first simply witnessed myself acting under their influence and made a conscious effort to override them before it finally became easier to step out of their influence. Today, they still occasionally catch up with me. As soon as I become aware of a driver influencing my behavior, I simply adjust my attitude.

The more we override our drivers, the more we are able to express how we truly feel and take action to get back to our inner balance, instead of numbing ourselves with food to avoid expressing anything. When we accept that we feel our emotions, we can welcome them when they arise. We can decide to express what we feel in a healthy way for us while still paying attention to the other person's emotions. Every time we are able to express our needs, we decrease our urge to eat as a way to deal with how we feel because our needs are not met.

Jump-Start

→ **Please describe a situation that activated your emotional eating response lately. What happened?**

→ **How did you feel?**

➜ **What did you need? Did you get it?**

➜ **How did you react, and what did you express?**

➜ **How did you let the other person know how you were feeling?**

➜ **What is something important that you have not allowed yourself to tell someone so far, and that you really need to let them know?**

➜ **In what area(s) of your life can you be less judgmental toward yourself?**

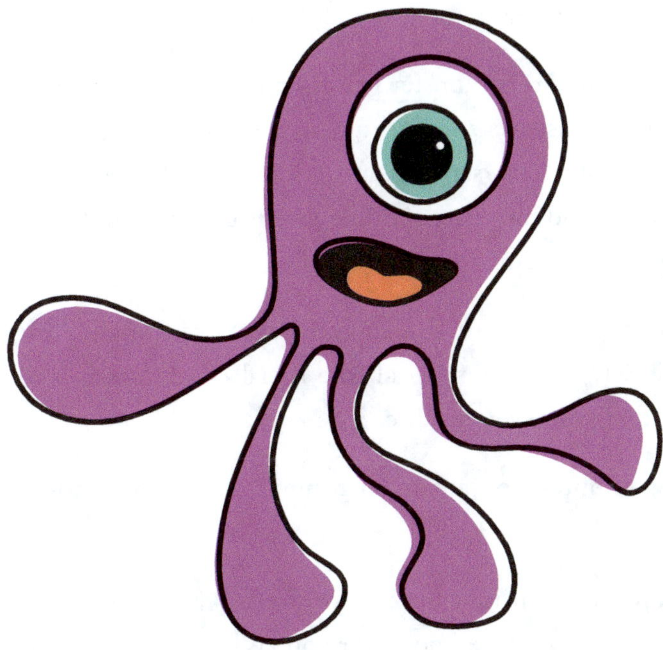

Thinking Outside the Box

Motion unleashes emotion. Unexpressed emotions are stuck energy in our bodies. Motion releases these energetic knots from our bodies. Whenever connecting with our emotions feels difficult or when we get upset, moving our bodies brings some relief and helps express our feelings.

This body-mind exercise is meant to help you release your suppressed emotions through your body and therefore significantly reduce your stress.

It is inspired by reactions and behavior young children use to release their own emotions. As they are still not "socially trained," they naturally express and instantly get rid of whatever they feel. After what may appear to adults to be a chaotic episode, they feel good again.

Please take twenty minutes alone in a room when you know you will not be disturbed, and get comfortable. Practice this exercise with the maximum comfortable intensity for you: be as intense as you can be without hurting yourself or your vocal cords or making a wrong move.

Stand up, with your arms alongside your body. Let your head fall forward, and close your eyes as you breathe in and out slowly a few times. Imagine you are a very mean and very scary monster.

Let yourself go as if you are a monster getting out of a space capsule after a very long space trip, only to discover strange humans staring at you. Open up your arms and make scary faces, use scary screams, weird sounds, and accentuated breathing. Open your eyes wide, and move around like a monster who would try to scare the imaginary people in the room where you are.

Let go of all the tension in your throat. Free your face, tongue, fingers, hands, arms, hips, legs, feet, and toes from all the social conditioning and emotional repression implied in your everyday life.

During these few minutes, you are an alien monster, free of all conformism and mental control.

Be as intense as you can without hurting yourself. Practice this exercise as long as you want and as long as it feels good for you. When you are done, slow down gradually and come back to your usual self.

→ **How are you feeling right after this exercise?**

If any emotion suddenly pops up, and you feel like crying, dancing, talking to someone who is not really there, venting about something, stomping your feet, or exploring any other physical manifestation, let it be, and even emphasize your movements if you can. This exercise is to bring your suppressed emotions closer to the surface; allow them to break free. Doing so will set you free too.

You can practice this exercise as often as you want to, especially after a stressful day.

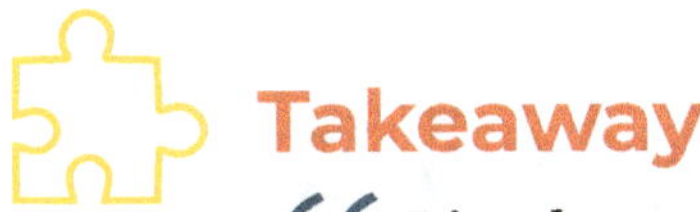

Takeaway

> *It's a lot easier to be angry at someone than it is to tell them you're hurt."*

—*Tom Gates*

You are already successful!

Congratulations! You made it through this important step. It was tough, but you pushed through it. Every time you engage in negative self-talk, please remember you've come this far, and there is no way you could have done this without willpower or a strong desire to bring positive and long-lasting change to your life.

In addition, you are probably not a total stranger to what we discussed in this chapter. That means you have been on your way to recovery for some time. Let's capitalize on your existing achievements and experience.

➔ **What have you already tried/started/accomplished in the area discussed in this chapter that previously worked/was a success/was promising?**

____

____

➔ **What happened to get you started?**

____

____

➔ **What was your recipe for success?**

____

____

➔ **How can you use this proven successful recipe today?**

____

____

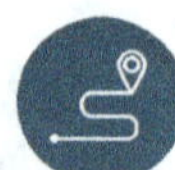 *Along the Path*

➜ **What have you been through while reading this chapter** *(what happened, how did you feel, what were your reactions, what important conversation did you have, did you have unusual dreams or body reactions/sensations)?*

➜ **What new perspective did you grasp in your relationship with food and with yourself or others or both?**

➜ **What new concept did you discover?**

➜ **What did you learn?**

➜ **What realization did you come to?**

➜ **What do you want to remember?**

 *Moving Forward*

WHAT WILL YOU DO LESS?

✖

✖

✖

WHAT WILL YOU STOP DOING?

✖

✖

✖

WHAT WILL YOU START DOING?

✓

✓

✓

WHAT WILL YOU DO MORE OF?

✓

✓

✓

→ **Which one of these decisions will be the easiest for you to apply right now?**

You may feel what you have discovered and processed during this chapter is enough for you to successfully impact your relationship with food. This is great, and you are ready to jump into the next change. You may also feel it would be useful for you to dig deeper and explore these topics or some related areas a little bit more. If you want to take your reflection process and experimentation one step further, do this exercise.

WHAT ASPECTS DO YOU WANT TO EXPLORE MORE?

HOW WILL YOU MAKE THIS EXPLORATION POSSIBLE?

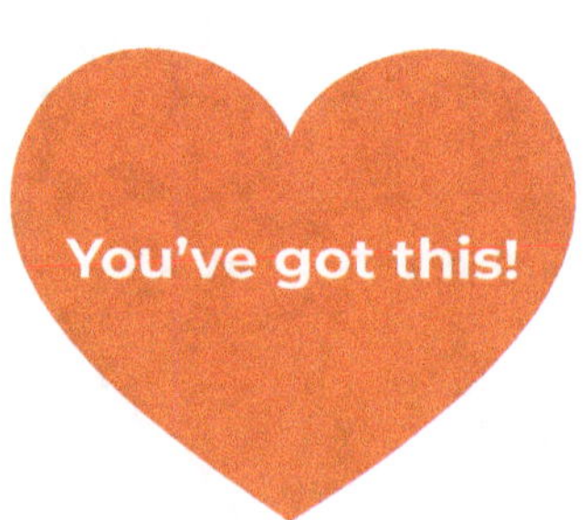

NOTES:

BEFORE YOU GO

Your Future Self
without Emotional Eating

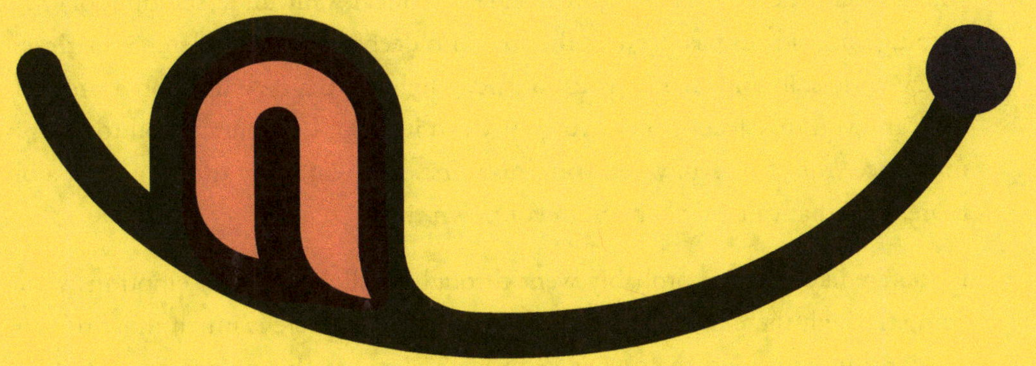

Your Future Self without Emotional Eating

Congratulations! You have completed the first book of the *Never Eat Your Emotions Again* series and the first part of your journey. The first step often is the most difficult to take, but here you are. You made it! It takes dedication and hard work to get where you are right now. You've done a great job, and you deserve to be proud of your accomplishments.

Remember, depending on how familiar you are with certain topics and how deeply you have already explored them (or not), you may need to go back to some chapters and give yourself more time to fully process them. That is perfectly fine and normal. If you feel right now that there may be something more to one of the steps you've already taken, you are free to study it again immediately.

If you feel ready to go ahead with the next part of your journey, please do.

And, if sometime later you feel like exploring again a topic you already covered, you are welcome to. Personal growth rarely is linear. Our understanding of what is going on inside us has to go further but also deeper to be complete. Sometimes, a new understanding later in your journey might shed a new light on a previous step, and you may feel the need to go back to it. If so, I encourage you to. This is not a race. You don't win when you finish first. You win every time you heal a bit more. And that can only happen in your own time.

If you are like me, you probably went through a roller coaster of emotions while going through these first steps. You also have realized there is much more to your relationship with food than what is on your plate. At this point, if you feel the need to ask a few questions, clarify something, or if you simply wish to share your testimonial, please reach out on social media. I would love to hear from you and how you are doing with your journey.

Instagram: Marion Holt (@nevereatyouremotionsagain)
instagram.com/nevereatyouremotionsagain/

Facebook: Marion Holt
facebook.com/profile.php?id=100061108901054

The emotional path I am taking you on is difficult, and I am aware of that. You might find some insight and additional emotional support from others who truly understand your journey in my free Facebook Support Group.

Facebook Support Group: Never Eat Your Emotions Again Network
facebook.com/groups/nevereatyouremotionsagain

You are now ready to take your recovery a step further. You may feel like jumping directly into one of the next books in the series, but you might also feel like you want to take a break and process what you have already been through. Both reactions are legitimate, and mostly related to your natural temper.

If you feel like digging deeper on your own into the topics of any chapter, you can explore the different options available on my website.

Explore: nevereatyouremotionsagain.com

If you would like to discuss a specific aspect of your recovery journey with me, please schedule a call.

Free Call: nevereatyouremotionsagain.com/free-call

Some of us need regular milestones to progressively integrate our discoveries, while others reflect on the path they walked only once they cross the finish line. Just listen to yourself, and give yourself what you need. If you feel like taking a break for a while, here is a little training that I like using myself, which you can easily add to your daily routine in the meantime.

Access my website and links using this QR code:

nevereatyouremotionsagain.com/links

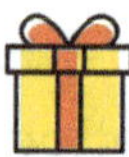

I have a gift for you.

Going through this book has been a difficult journey, and you made it. To celebrate your accomplishment, I would like to offer you a metaphoric gift.

I am gifting you a trip to your favorite amusement park to play with your inner child.

Please take a moment to write down where you go together, how you feel, what activities you do together, how much fun you have, what you talk about—everything to describe how your day goes and how much you enjoy it.

When you're done, take a few minutes to sit with your feelings and your inner child. Keep your writings about that day, and every time you feel disconnected from yourself or your inner child, go back to the amusement park with them.

With this exercise, you train yourself to experience a deeper connection with your inner child, allowing them to express themselves more freely. You also get used to feeling the difference between moments when you are well-connected to yourself and your emotions and when you are not. The more you consciously create moments to connect with your inner child, the easier it will become to let your true self shine.

If this is the first book you have read in this series, please check out the contents of the next books. See what is waiting for you, and decide the next step you want to take. I am so proud of you! Keep up the good work. Remember...

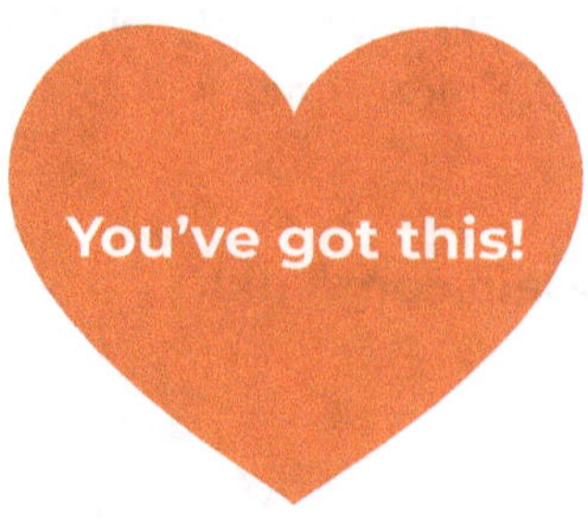

A peek at what lies ahead:

Never Eat Your Emotions Again, Book 2

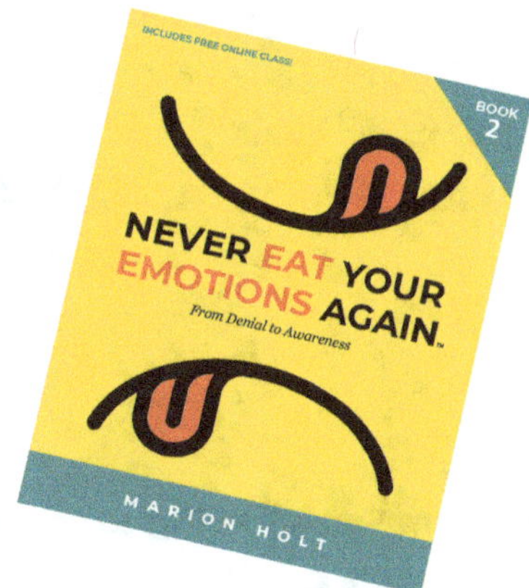

Never Eat Your Emotions Again, Book 3

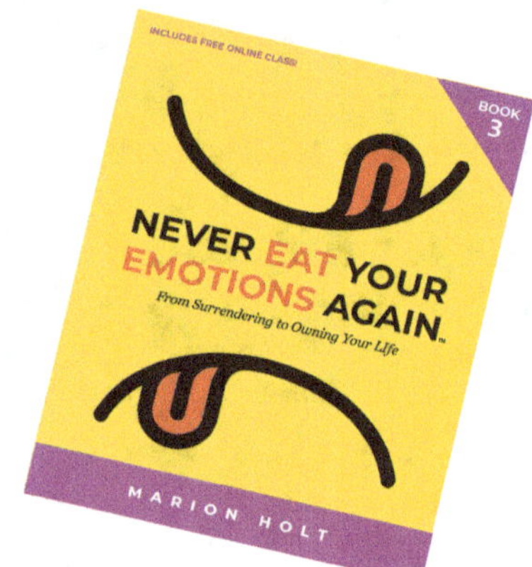

Part V: From Surrendering to Owning Your Life

Step 13: Choose to Live

You Deserve More Than the Life You Allow Yourself to Live

- The Challenge: Guilt Complex and Internalized Shame
- How to Take Your Life Back

Step 14: Defeat Your Repetition Compulsion

You Are More Than What Happened to You

- The Challenge: Unaddressed Trauma
- How to Break Patterns that No Longer Serve You

Step 15: Learn from Your Relapses

You Don't Fail until You Stop Trying

- The Challenge: Learned Helplessness
- How to Unlearn Learned Helplessness

Part VI: Eureka! I Found Me!

Step 16: Restore Fair Relationships

Your Worth and What You Provide to Others Are Not Tied Together

- The Challenge: Parentification
- How to Build Relationships Where Your Needs Are Met

Step 17: Be Unapologetically Who You Are

You Are You, and You Are Enough

- The Challenge: Personality Masking
- How to Embrace Your Personal Power

Step 18: Love Yourself

Self-Love Does Not Depend on the Way You Look or How Much You Eat

- The Challenge: Low Self-Esteem
- How to Heal Your Conditional-Love Scars

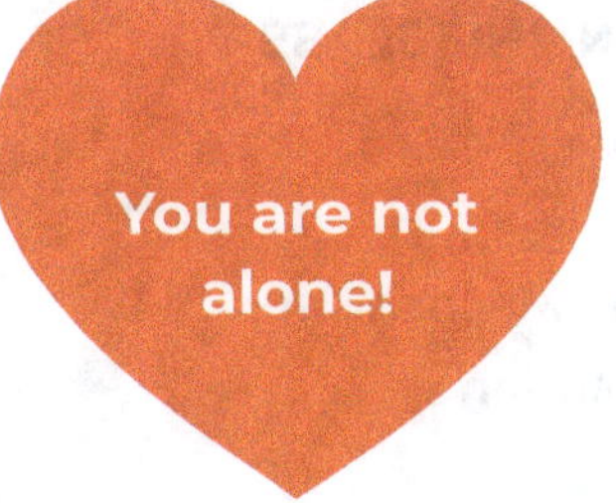
You are not
alone!

Thank You for reading
NEVER EAT YOUR EMOTIONS AGAIN, Book 1

If you enjoyed the book, I would very much appreciate it if you would leave a review on Amazon, Goodreads, BookBub, or the platform you used. Your review will guide other emotional eaters toward what they can expect from this book and whether it matches their needs.

I hope you will continue your recovery journey with Book 2, and in the meanwhile, you can access some additional free online classes here, including: three videos, three PDF lessons, three workbooks, and one quiz.

ONLINE CLASS: WHAT EMOTIONAL EATING REALLY IS

**YOUR FREE SUPPORTIVE ONLINE CLASS
INCLUDES THREE LESSONS:**

→ The Many Faces of Emotional Eating
→ Emotional Eating as a Coping Mechanism
→ Emotional Eating as a Compulsion

GET YOUR FREE ACCESS TO:

→ 3 PDF lessons
→ 3 workbooks

Open your welcome gift now!
nevereatyouremotionsagain.com/links

ONLINE CLASSES AND SIGNATURE PROGRAM

Not everybody has the same learning style. If you feel like reviewing or digging deeper into any chapter of any of the three books in the series, you can access my online classes here:

nevereatyouremotionsagain.com/classes

I put a special emphasis on meeting everybody's needs to the closest and to the fullest way possible. That's why my online classes are *à la carte.* You can choose to:

➔   **Access one specific class at a time, with supporting PDFs, videos, workbooks, and quizzes. You can check out all the classes available here:** nevereatyouremotionsagain.com/classes

Or. . .

➔ **Join my signature program, that will give you access to all the steps, with all the supporting materials. It also includes several individual coaching sessions to work one-on-one with me and unlock some very specific situations you might be faced with on your recovery journey. In addition, you will join my private community and be able to discuss and share what you are going through with your peers, in the same program, and benefit from their experience. You can get more information about my signature program here:** nevereatyouremotionsagain.com/program

My goal is to provide everything you need to see you succeed on your journey. You can do this!

These links are all accessible via the website:
nevereatyouremotionsagain.com/links

RESOURCES

If you would like to read more (and I know you will), I recommend the following resources.

Books

Anderson, S. (2015). *Taming your outer child: Overcoming self-sabotage and healing from abandonment.* New World Library.

Bandura, A. (1997). *Self-efficacy, the exercise of control.* Freeman.

Berne E. (1996). *Games people play: The basic handbook of transactional analysis.* Ballantine Books.

Bernier, L., & Lenghan, R. (2016). *The little stick figures technique by Jacques Martel. (French ed.).* New Leaf Distributing Co Inc.

Blackman, J. S. (2003). *101 defenses: How the mind shields itself.* Routledge.

Bourbeau, L. (2002). *Heal your wounds and find your true self.* Lotus Press.

Bowlby, J. (2008). *A secure base: Parent-child attachment and healthy human development.* Basic Books.

Bradshaw, J. (2005). *Healing the shame that binds you.* Health Communications Inc.

Bradshaw, J. (2013). *Homecoming: Reclaiming and championing your inner child.* Bantam.

Braiker, H. B. (2003). *Who's pulling your strings? How to break the cycle of manipulation and regain control of your life.* McGraw-Hill.

Brown, B. (2007). *I thought it was just me (but it isn't): Making the journey from "what will people think?" to "I am enough."* Avery.

Burgo, J. (2012). *Why do I do that? Psychological defense mechanisms and the hidden ways they shape our lives.* New Rise Press.

Burke Harris, N. (2019). *The deepest well: Healing the long-term effects of childhood adversity.* Mariner Books.

Burns, D. D. (2012). *Feeling good, the new mood therapy: The clinically proven drug-free treatment for depression.* Harper.

Cangelosi, James S. (2013). *Classroom Management Strategies: Gaining and maintaining students' cooperation.* John Wiley & Sons.

Carlson, N. R., Miller, H. L., Heth, D. S., Donahoe, J. W., & Martin, G. N. (2007). *Psychology: The science of behavior (7th ed.).* Pearson Education Canada.

Chase, N. D. (1999). *Burdened children: Theory, research, and treatment of parentification.* SAGE Publications, Inc.

Cottone, P., Sabino, V., Moore, C.F., & Koob, G. F. (2019). *Compulsive eating behavior and food addiction: Emerging pathological constructs.* Academic Press.

Cottraux, J. (2001). *La répétition des scénarios de vie: Demain est une autre histoire.* [Life scenarios repetitions: tomorrow's another day.] Jacob.

Cuddy, A. (2018). *Presence: Bringing your boldest self to your biggest challenges.* Little, Brown Spark.

Cudney, M., & Hardy, R. E. (2010). *Self-defeating behaviors: Free yourself from the habits, compulsions, feelings and attitudes that hold you back.* HarperOne.

Denborough, D. (2014). *Retelling the stories of our lives: Everyday narrative therapy to draw inspiration and transform experience.* W. W. Norton & Company.

Engel, B. (2003). *The emotionally abusive relationship: How to stop being abused and how to stop abusing.* Wiley.

Forsyth, J.P., & Eifert, G. H. (2016). *The mindfulness and acceptance workbook for anxiety.* New Harbinger Publications.

Gibson, L. C. (2015). *Adult children of emotionally immature parents: How to heal from distant, rejecting or self-involved parents.* New Harbinger Publications.

Gross, J. J. (2014). *Handbook of Emotion Regulation.* Guilford.

Hay, L. (2016). *Mirror work: 21 days to heal your life.* Hay House Inc.

Hill, C. (2021). *Healthy boundaries: How to set strong boundaries, say no without guilt, and maintain good relationships with your parents, family, and friends.* Independently published.

Hohmann, L. (2006). *Innovation games: Creating breakthrough products through collaborative play.* Addison-Wesley Professional.

Kahler, T. (2008). *The process therapy model: The six personality types with adaptations.* Taibi Kahler Associates, Inc.

Kallel, S., & Masselot, O. (2018). *Le leadership du coeur: Les 4 postures des nouveaux leaders. [Leadership of the heart: the new leaders 4 stances.]* Gereso.

Kishimi, I., & Koga, F. (2018). *The courage to be disliked.* Atria Books.

Levin, N. (2020). *Setting boundaries will set you free: The ultimate guide to telling the truth, creating connection, and finding freedom.* Hay House Inc.

Levine, P. A. (1997). *Waking the Tiger: Healing Trauma.* North Atlantic Books

McKay, M. (2016). *Self-esteem: A proven program of cognitive techniques for assessing, improving, and maintaining your self-esteem.* New Harbinger Publications.

McLaren, K. (2010). *The language of emotions: What your feelings are trying to tell you.* Sounds True Publishing.

Middelton-Moz, J. (1990). *Shame & guilt, masters of disguise.* Health Communications Inc.

Miller, A. (2004). *Notre corps ne ment jamais. [Our body never lies.]* Flammarion.

Morgan, O. (2019). *Addiction, attachment, trauma and recovery: The power of connection.* W.W. Norton & Company.

Napper, P., and Rao, A. (2019). The power of agency: The 7 principles to conquer obstacles, make effective *decisions, and create a life on your own terms.* St. Martin's Press.

Peterson, C., Maier, S. F., & Seligman, M. E. P. (1995). *Learned helplessness: A theory for the age of personal control.* Oxford University Press.

Price, D. (2021). *Laziness does not exist.* Atria Books.

Scherrer, D. (2018). *Accompagner avec l'arbre de vie: Une pratique narrative pour restaurer l'estime de soi. [The tree of life: a narrative therapy practice to restore self-esteem.]* Intereditions.

Schiraldi, G.R. (2021). *The adverse childhood experiences recovery workbook: Heal the hidden wounds from childhood affecting your mental and physical health (workbook ed.).* New Harbinger Publications.

Schwartz, A. (2017). *Complex PTSD workbook: A mind-body approach to regaining emotional control and becoming whole.* Althea Press.

Séméria, E. (2018). *Le harcèlement fusionnel, les ressorts cachés de la dépendance affective.* [Fusional harassment, the hidden motives of emotional dependence.] Albin Michel.

Snel, E. (2019). *Proche, mais pas trop.* [Close, but not too close.] Arènes.

Tal Schaller, C., & Razanamahay-Schaller, J. (2010). *Vivre les émotions avec son corps : Se libérer des tensions pour vivre heureux.* [Experience emotions through the body.]

Thayer, R. (2001). *How people regulate mood with food and exercise.* Oxford University Press.

Van der Kolk, B. (2015). *The body keeps the score: Brain, mind and body in the healing of trauma.* Penguin Books.

Watzlavick, P., Weakland, J. H., & Fisch, R. (2011). *Change: Principles of problem formation and problem resolution.* W. W. Norton & Company.

Williamson, M., (1996). *A return to love. Reflections on the principles of a course in miracles.* HarperOne. Reissued Edition.

Wolynn, M. (2017). *It didn't start with you: How inherited family trauma shapes who we are and how to end the cycle.* Penguin Life.

Young, J. E., Klosko, J. S., & Weishaar, M. E. (2006). *Schema therapy: A practitioner's guide.* Guilford Press.

Articles

Arnow, B., Kenardy, J., & Agras, W. S. (1995). The emotional eating scale: The development of a measure to assess coping with negative affect by eating. *The International Journal of Eating Disorders, 18*(1), 79–90. The emotional eating scale: The development of a measure to assess coping with negative affect by eating - Arnow - 1995 - International Journal of Eating Disorders - Wiley Online Library

Babbel, S. (n.d.). The connection between emotional stress, trauma & physical pain. *Dr. Susanne Babbel.* The Connections Between Emotional Stress, Trauma & Physical Pain — Dr. Susanne Babbel (drbabbel.com)

Bastian, B., Jetten, J., & Fasoli, F. (2011). Cleansing the soul by hurting the flesh: The guilt-reducing effect of pain. *Psychological Science, 22*(3), 334–335. https://doi.org/10.1177/0956797610397058

Blundell, A. (2022, October 18). Healthy Boundaries—12 signs you lack them (and why you need them). *Harley Therapy Counselling Blog.* https://www.harleytherapy.co.uk/counselling/healthy-boundaries.htm

Blundell, A. (2022, May 3). The victim mentality: What it is and why you use it. *Harley Therapy Counselling Blog.* https://www.harleytherapy.co.uk/counselling/victim-mentality.htm

Bourdin, D. (2016). *La culpabilité d'exister, culpabilité primaire.* [Guilty of Existing, Primary Guilt] Société Psychanalytique de Paris. https://www.spp.asso.fr/textes/textes-et-conferences/conferences-de-sainte-anne/la-culpabilite-dexister-culpabilite-primaire/

Brennan, C. (2013, March 8). The broken bowl project. The Broken Bowl Project | christabrennan (wordpress.com)

Brewerton, T. D. (2007). Eating disorders, trauma, and comorbidity: Focus on PTSD. *Eating Disorders, 15*(4), 285–304. Eating Disorders, Trauma, and Comorbidity: Focus on PTSD: Eating Disorders: Vol 15, No 4 (tandfonline.com)

Brown, B. (2012). *Listening to Shame* [Video]. TED Conferences. https://www.ted.com/talks/ brene_brown_listening_to_shame

Brown, B. (2013, January 15). Shame vs. guilt. *Brené Brown.* https://brenebrown.com/ blog/2013/01/14/shame-v-guilt

Callan, M. J., Kay, A. C., & Dawtry, R. J. (2014). Making sense of misfortune: Deservingness, self-esteem, and patterns of self-defeat. *Journal of Personality and Social Psychology, 107*(1), 142–162. Making sense of misfortune: Deservingness, self-esteem, and patterns of self-defeat. (apa.org)

Cash, T. F., Fleming, E. C., Alindogan, J., Steadman, L., & Whitehead, A. (2002). Beyond body image as a trait: The development and validation of the body image states scale. E*ating Disorders: The Journal of Treatment & Prevention, 10*(2), 103–113. Beyond Body Image as a Trait: The Development and Validation of the Body Image States Scale: Eating Disorders: Vol 10, No 2 (tandfonline.com)

Dunkley, D. M., Masheb, R. M., & Grilo, C. M. (2010). Childhood maltreatment, depressive symptoms, and body dissatisfaction in patients with binge eating disorder: the mediating role of self-criticism. *The International Journal of Eating Disorders, 43*(3), 274–281. Childhood maltreatment, depressive symptoms, and body dissatisfaction in patients with binge eating disorder: The mediating role of self-criticism - Dunkley - 2010 - International Journal of Eating Disorders - Wiley Online Library

Fielding, L. (2015, October 20). Listening to Your Authentic Self: The purpose of emotions. *HuffPost.* https://www.huffpost.com/entry/finding-your-authentic-pu_b_8342280

Fletcher, J. (2022, October 27). 11 personality masks we wear. *PsychCentral.com.* https://psychcentral. com/health/the-masks-we-wear

Fletcher, P. C., & Kenny, P. J. (2018). Food addiction: A valid concept? *Neuropsychopharmacology: Official Publication of the American College of Neuropsychopharmacology, 43*(13), 2506–2513. Food addiction: a valid concept? | Neuropsychopharmacology (nature.com)

Gilman, J. (2021). The five signs of emotional suffering. *Healthy365 Connection Center.* The Five Signs of Emotional Suffering - BeHealthy365

Guarino, G. M. (2021). Emotions worksheets. *Psych Point.* https://www.psychpoint.com/worksheets/ emotions-worksheets

Hebebrand, J., Albayrak, Ö., Adan, R., Antel, J., Dieguez, C., de Jong, J., Leng, G., Menzies, J., Mercer, J. G., Murphy, M., van der Plasse, G., & Dickson, S. L. (2014). "Eating addiction", rather than "food addiction", better captures addictive-like eating behavior. *Neuroscience and Biobehavioral Reviews, 47,* 295–306. "Eating addiction", rather than "food addiction", better captures addictive-like eating behavior - ScienceDirect

Katz, J., Petracca, M., & Rabinowitz, J. (2009). A retrospective study of daughters' emotional role reversal with parents, attachment anxiety, excessive reassurance-seeking, and depressive symptoms. *American Journal of Family Therapy, 37*(3), 185–195. A Retrospective Study of Daughters' Emotional Role Reversal with Parents, Attachment Anxiety, Excessive Reassurance-Seeking, and Depressive Symptoms: The American Journal of Family Therapy: Vol 37, No 3 (tandfonline.com)

Lisitsa, E. (2013). Manage conflict: Identifying your triggers. *Gottman Institute.* https://www.gottman. com/blog/manage-conflict-triggers/

Liu, C., & Bates, T. C. (2014). The structure of attributional style: Cognitive styles and optimism–pessimism bias in the attributional style questionnaire. *Personality and Individual Differences, 66,* 79–85. The structure of attributional style: Cognitive styles and optimism–pessimism bias in the Attributional Style Questionnaire - ScienceDirect

Mariage, A., Cuynet, P., & Carvelli-Roussel, G. (2005). L'obésité chez l'adulte à l'épreuve du Rorschach. [Testing adult obesity with Rorschach.] *Bulletin de psychologie, 476,* 207–219. L'obésité chez l'adulte à l'épreuve du Rorschach | Cairn.info

Maté, G. (07-08/2017). The addict in all of us. *Psychotherapy Networker.* The Addict in All of Us (psychotherapynetworker.org)

McNeel, J.R., (2010). Understanding the power of injunctive messages and how they are resolved in redecision therapy. *Transactional Analysis Journal, 40*(2), 159–169. Understanding the Power of Injunctive Messages and How They are Resolved in Redecision Therapy: Transactional Analysis Journal: Vol 40, No 2 (tandfonline.com)

Mitchell, K. S., Mazzeo, S. E., Schlesinger, M. R., Brewerton, T. D., & Smith, B. N. (2012). Comorbidity of partial and subthreshold ptsd among men and women with eating disorders in the national comorbidity survey-replication study. *The International Journal of Eating Disorders, 45*(3), 307–315. Comorbidity of partial and subthreshold ptsd among men and women with eating disorders in the national comorbidity survey-replication study - Mitchell - 2012 - International Journal of Eating Disorders - Wiley Online Library

Monjauze, M. (2001). Psychanalyse de l'« objet ». « Objet-drogue », « objet-alcool ». [Psychoanalysis of the "object". "Drug-object", "alcool-object".] *Le Carnet PSY, 61,* 17–22. Psychanalyse de l'« objet ». « Objet-drogue », « objet-alcool » | Cairn.info

Orbach, I., Mikulincer, M., Gilboa-Schechtman, E., & Sirota, P. (2003). Mental pain and its relationship to suicidality and life meaning. *Suicide & Life-Threatening Behavior, 33*(3), 231–241. Mental Pain and Its Relationship to Suicidality and Life Meaning - Orbach - 2003 - Suicide and Life-Threatening Behavior - Wiley Online Library

Peterson, T. J. (2016, July 7). Guilt: A distressing effect of anxiety. *Healthy Place.* https://www.healthyplace.com/blogs/anxiety-schmanxiety/2016/07/guilt-a-distressing-effect-of-anxiety

PsychologyToday.com Staff. (n.d.). *Emotion Regulation.* Emotion Regulation | Psychology Today

Sack, M., Boroske-Leiner, K., & Lahmann, C. (2010). Association of nonsexual and sexual traumatizations with body image and psychosomatic symptoms in psychosomatic outpatients. *General Hospital Psychiatry, 32*(3), 315–320. Association of nonsexual and sexual traumatizations with body image and psychosomatic symptoms in psychosomatic outpatients - ScienceDirect

Sincero, S. M. (2011). *Operant Conditioning.* Retrieved Oct. 15, 2022 from Explorable.com. https://explorable.com/operant-conditioning

Taylor, T. F. (2015). The influence of shame on posttrauma disorders: Have we failed to see the obvious? *European Journal of Psychotraumatology, 6*(1), 28847. Full article: The influence of shame on posttrauma disorders: have we failed to see the obvious? (tandfonline.com)

Travis, A. C., Pawa, S., LeBlanc, J. K., & Rogers, A. I. (2011). Denial: What is it, how do we recognize it, and what should we do about it? *The American Journal of Gastroenterology, 106*(6), 1028–1030. Denial: What Is It, How Do We Recognize It, and What Should... : Official journal of the American College of Gastroenterology | ACG (lww.com)

Tsakiris, M., Schütz-Bosbach, S., & Gallagher, S. (2007). On agency and body-ownership: Phenomenological and neurocognitive reflections. *Consciousness and Cognition, 16*(3), 645–660. On agency and body-ownership: Phenomenological and neurocognitive reflections - ScienceDirect

Turton, R., Chami, R., & Treasure, J. (2017). Emotional eating, binge eating and animal models of binge-type eating disorders. *Current obesity reports, 6*(2), 217–228. Emotional Eating, Binge Eating and Animal Models of Binge-Type Eating Disorders | SpringerLink

Wikipedia (2022) Prentification. Parentification - Wikipedia

Wood, A. M., Linley, A. P., Maltby, J., Baliousis, M., & Joseph, S. (2008). The authentic personality: A theoretical and empirical conceptualization and the development of the authenticity scale. *Journal of Counseling Psychology, 55*(3), 385–399. Sci-Hub | The authentic personality: A theoretical and empirical conceptualization and the development of the Authenticity Scale. Journal of Counseling Psychology, 55(3), 385–399 | 10.1037/0022-0167.55.3.385

Wood, J. V., Heimpel, S. A., Manwell, L. A., & Whittington, E. J. (2009). This mood is familiar and I don't deserve to feel better anyway: Mechanisms underlying self-esteem differences in motivation to repair sad moods. *Journal of personality and social psychology, 96*(2), 363–380. This mood is familiar, and I don't deserve to feel better anyway: mechanisms underlying self-esteem differences in motivation to repair sad moods - PubMed (nih.gov)

World Health Organization Team. (2020). Adverse Childhood Experiences International Questionnaire (ACE-IQ). https://www.who.int/publications/m/item/adverse-childhood-experiences-international-questionnaire-(ace-iq)

ACKNOWLEDGMENTS

I thought writing a book was a solitary task. I was wrong. From people who helped shape the experience I poured into this book, to those who shared their own experience; from people who helped make this combination of tumultuous thoughts look appealing and professional, to those who endured my writer's mood shifts and never-ending existential questions; from people who encouraged me to persevere finishing a series that could help others, to those who lifted me up when I did not believe in myself, I was never alone. Writing this book was a team effort, and I would like to thank the following:

My husband, Jim, who thought I was embarking on a one-year project that turned into four, yet you never stopped believing in me. You were the only one I trusted enough to take the first look at my manuscript. You shared your honest thoughts without hurting my feelings and helped my project grow better. From day one, you have allowed me to be 100 percent myself in your eyes and still feel loved. None of this would have been possible without you. Je t'aime mon amour.

Becky Yates, who went in-depth into my manuscript, and gave me some precious feedback. You allowed me to make this book a better experience for the readers. I couldn't have asked for a better sister-in-law.

Candace Johnson, my editor, who patiently and brilliantly fixed my non-native English prose, without ever distorting my thoughts.

Anj Riffel, my graphic designer, who made me feel heard, and walked me through my doubts and tough choices with kindness and empathy. Her cover design gives an unforgettable look to this series and her interior design makes working through an emotional process fun and heartwarming.

Agnès Cart-Lamy, who coached me through my moments of self-doubt all along the writing process and allowed me to embrace several perspectives. No matter how agitated, defeated, or lost I felt at the beginning of a talk with you, I ended every single conversation feeling anchored, at peace, and ready to keep going. You are one of the best coaches I've ever worked with, and your friendship is so precious to me.

Julien Bodin, another excellent coach, who facilitated the quick start of my emotional eating recovery journey and the writing of this book when my fears were holding me back. You are the friend I call when I need some tough love.

Amélie Borgniat, certified expert in traditional Chinese medicine, who gave me the best acupuncture sessions I have ever had. She now guides me through efficient self-relief practice from across the ocean, when I am stuck in overdrive, or when my energy level crashes. Thank you for the authenticity of your friendship. Wherever our respective paths take us, I know you will always be there.

Pastor Mike Gibson, who counseled me at a painful time during my recovery journey. You helped me go through some difficult realizations and tough choices and never once judged me.

Leigh Harris, who allowed me to work out with other women in a safe, fun, and never judgmental environment when I was too insecure to set foot in a fitness class.

All the women working out with me, contributing to make it a fellowship and fun experience instead of a painful chore, including Ashley, Barbara, Siobhan, Vicky, Paula, Deborah, Melody, Anita, Darlene, Maria, and Katie.

Brian Harris, web designer, who graciously helped me through building a website and out of the biggest mistakes—like deleting my front page. Your input was invaluable. Knowing you had my back allowed me to step way out of my comfort zone.

Kevin Thornton, who made me stretch muscles I never knew I had. Your ability to meet everyone at the physical level they are and provide an efficient workout designed to respect individual abilities is remarkable.

Jeanne Gray-Carr, an experienced coach who introduced me to the world of coaching in the mid-South. Your guidance helped me get started.

Jana Cardona, a talented coach and former executive director in Business Network International (BNI). You showed me how to start a business in the United States and the standards of referrals in the mid-South.

Michel Zylbermann, CEO of Erudia, and Olivier Masselot and Samy Kallel, co-creators of "NeuroSensorial Intelligence" and the "Leadership of the Heart." Your training led me into coaching and improved my abilities.

The Great Banquet of the Mid-South organization, their team members, and volunteers at the time I participated, including Kellie Evins, Kathy Downen, Stephanie Russell, Paula Denbow, Sylvia Henry, Mona Arick, Leslie King, Carrie Whaley, Diann White, Jordan Walston, and Nicole Powell. I had a great spiritual experience and was able to finally let go of a difficult matter I did not have control over. I found precious fellowship and made new friendships during this retreat. All of you contributed to this unique experience and my spiritual growth.

Celebrate Recovery and Stacy and Steve, the leaders of my chapter at the time I attended. Though I did not attend many sessions, it was enough to notice the remarkable job you both did as leaders of this group. You and all the participants helped me realize that even though some people choose to cope with various substances or behaviors when I choose food, we are all equal, and we are all turning to something because we are in pain and hurt in the same way.

All my friends, including Marc Quetel and Anne-Lise Burgert, who were my friends before my recovery journey, who stuck with me during the process, and who are still my friends today, accepting and loving the "new me." Even if there is an ocean between us now, my world would not be the same without your friendship.

All my clients, whose trust honors me, and whose stories immensely contributed to this book.

About the Author

Marion Holt is a certified professional coach from the Université Catholique de l'Ouest in Angers, France, and holds a DISC behavior assessment certification. She is an emotional eater. She has struggled multiple times to lose weight, focusing exclusively on food, eating habits, and exercise. Marion failed every attempt and ended up affected by severe obesity. She sought professional and medical help but was unsuccessful. For years, she believed her weight loss was a lost cause.

Marion was able to change her relationship with food when she realized it was based on an emotional coping mechanism. Using her behavioral expertise, she addressed the root causes of her way of eating, made the necessary changes in her life, and finally lost weight.

Marion now offers to others in the same situation the appropriate help she sought but could never find. She created a process to break free from emotional eating based both on her coaching expertise and her personal experience of emotional eating recovery. She helps her clients by targeting the underlying reasons why they eat their emotions and helps them toward building a life where they don't need the comfort of food anymore.

With the series *Never Eat Your Emotions Again,* she shares her emotional eating recovery process with everyone who struggles to achieve a healthy relationship with food.

Before specializing in emotional eating recovery, Marion graduated from law school, the prestigious HEC School of Management in Paris, France, and worked in the corporate world internationally. She now lives with her husband in Tennessee. Going from "city girl" to "farm girl" was a journey in itself. Every day now starts with gathering eggs, and she enjoys taking care of her horses, cats, dogs, numerous chickens, and occasional visiting ducks and geese.

Find out more about Marion Holt
and her coaching programs at:

nevereatyouremotionsagain.com

Connect with Marion:

Instagram:

Marion Holt (@nevereatyouremotionsagain)

instagram.com/nevereatyouremotionsagain/

Facebook:

Marion Holt

facebook.com/profile.php?id=100061108901054

Facebook Support Group:

Never Eat Your Emotions Again Network

facebook.com/groups/nevereatyouremotionsagain

Subscribe to her free monthly email newsletter and get tips to help your journey be successful:

subscribepage.com/neyeanewsletter

Access all links here:

nevereatyouremotionsagain.com/links